Intravenous
Therapy
A Guide to
Quality Care

Intravenous
Therapy
A Guide to
Quality Care

Connie White Delaney, Ph.D., R.N.
Assistant Professor
College of Nursing
The University of Iowa

Mary Lou Lauer, B.S., M.A.
Doctoral Candidate
The University of Iowa

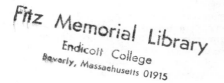

J. B. Lippincott Company Philadelphia
London Mexico City New York
St. Louis São Paulo Sydney

Sponsoring Editor: Diana Intenzo
Indexer: Maria Coughlin
Designer: Anne O'Donnell
Design Coordinator: Caren Erlichman
Production Manager: Carol A. Florence
Production Coordinator: Barney Fernandes
Compositor: Bi-Comp, Inc.
Printer/Binder: R. R. Donnelly & Sons Company

6   5   4   3   2   1

Library of Congress Cataloging-in-Publication Data

Delaney, Connie White.
  Intravenous therapy.

  Includes bibliography and index.
  1. Intravenous therapy. 2. Nursing. I. Lauer,
Mary Lou. II. Title. [DNLM: 1. Infusions, Parenteral—
handbooks.   2. Parenteral Feeding—handbooks.
WB 39 D337i] RM170.D45 1988   615.8'55   87-17009
ISBN 0-397-54617-3

Any procedure or practice described in this book should be applied by the health-care practitioner under appropriate supervision in accordance with professional standards of care used with regard to the unique circumstances that apply in each practice situation. Care has been taken to confirm the accuracy of information presented and to describe generally accepted practices. However, the authors, editors, and publisher cannot accept any responsibility for errors or omissions or for consequences from application of the information in this book and make no warranty, express or implied, with respect to the contents of the book.

Every effort has been made to ensure drug selections and dosages are in accordance with current recommendations and practice. Because of ongoing research, changes in government regulations, and the constant flow of information on drug therapy, reactions, and interactions, the reader is cautioned to check the package insert for each drug for indications, dosages, warnings, and precautions, particularly if the drug is new or infrequently used.

To those students and practitioners
dedicated to providing intravenous therapy
that focuses on the sensitivity
and wholeness of the art
as well as the breadth and depth
of the science.

Preface

Intravenous therapy has become a major component of patient care in the hospital, nursing home, and clinic settings, as well as home environments. Approximately 17 to 24 million hospitalized patients alone experienced at least one intravascular device insertion (NITA, 1986). Numerous infusates—including medications, blood products, and nutritional supplements—are administered through peripheral and/or central sites, utilizing a variety of infusion devices. A further look at this therapy reveals some of the risks involved. Each year 1.3 million patients experience intravenous infusion phlebitis; 35,000 patients experience septicemia; 3,000 patients may die as a result of complications related to blood products (Turco, 1983).

Students and practitioners must recognize that intravenous therapy is an area of continuing growth and an area subject to increasing morbidity and mortality. Promoting continued growth in practitioner expertise in administration techniques and prevention of complications is essential. Refinement of administration and monitoring practices will also encourage the practitioners to meet the need for financial accountability in these days of close scrutiny of expenses and emphasis on shorter patient stays.

An adequate intravenous therapy knowledge base requires incorporation of information from many areas, including anatomy, physiology, mathematics, physics, chemistry, histology, microbiology, and nursing. Synthesis of these areas promotes application of up-to-date, scientifically based nursing interventions. Due to time limitations nurse educators, regardless of program type or

level, are unable to devote large blocks of time to literature reviews and instruction in this area. Likewise staff
development and continuing education personnel have
limited time to devote to the area of intravenous therapy.

This concise yet comprehensive IV therapy handbook
provides the synthesis required. Designed for students,
practitioners, and educators in nursing programs, staff
development, and continuing education, this practical,
well-documented IV therapy handbook translates information and data from other disciplines into practical
knowledge and meaningful, sound interventions. The
nursing process provides the organizing framework for
much of the content. The inclusion of procedures facilitates applications. Referencing from pertinent research
validates the content. Since current nursing practices
may be challenged, change may result from use of this
resource.

The handbook is organized into six units.

Unit I: Foundations of Intravenous Therapy

The purpose of this unit is to provide a comprehensive,
concise foundation of background information that will
promote understanding and implementation of effective,
sound interventions in intravenous therapy. Chapter 1
contains a review of the physiological concepts of fluids
and electrolytes in the balanced state, including normal
body water distribution and the mechanisms that control
it; the concept and related assessment of acid/base balance; assessment of fluid imbalances with emphasis on
numerous physical and behavioral parameters and laboratory tests. Chapter 2 presents the rationale for fluid
replacement. A description of each infusate type is included along with suggestions and indications for use during specific imbalances. This information provides a basis
for nursing judgments related to assessment and evaluation of fluid therapy. Chapter 3 provides an overview of
IV equipment; emphasis is placed on specific equipment
characteristics that have ramifications for nursing inter-

ventions and complications. Chapter 4 includes a comprehensive outline of the flow properties of the intravenous gravity flow system and the venous system. Emphasis throughout is placed on those characteristics that have a major, direct impact on nursing interventions and/or the development of complications.

Unit II: Nursing Interventions: Techniques and Procedures of Intravenous Therapy

The purpose of this unit is to comprehensively discuss nursing interventions related to initiating, maintaining, and discontinuing intravascular therapy in adults, children, and the elderly. Nursing actions include diagnostic, therapeutic and educational interventions. Procedural outlines are included. Chapter 5 provides a step-by-step outline for initiating therapy. Chapter 6 outlines safe, appropriate nursing interventions for maintaining and discontinuing therapy; procedures and charting guidelines are integrated. Chapter 7 lends itself to special infusion situations including the uses, advantages, disadvantages, and nursing interventions for starting, maintaining, and discontinuing heparin locks; physiological and psychological implications, equipment needs, nursing interventions, and complications specific to the pediatric patient; and physical and psychological changes of aging, equipment implications, nursing interventions, and complications specific to the elderly patient.

Unit III: Complications of Intravenous Therapy

This unit comprehensively lists and describes over thirty complications that occur during and as a result of intravenous therapy. Each complication is discussed according to causes, how the nurse can anticipate and recognize the complication and interventions that can be used to treat and, more important, prevent the complication. Chapter 8 concerns localized complications, whereas Chapter 9 describes those that are systemic.

Unit IV: Parenteral Nutrition

A discussion of total parenteral nutrition (TPN) is provided in this unit. Chapter 10 briefly outlines the basics of nutrition and emphasizes the assessment of nutritional status. It culminates in identification of criteria for selection of TPN candidates. Chapter 11 describes nursing interventions for TPN administration. Chapter 12 focuses on mechanical, infectious, and metabolic complications of parenteral nutrition.

Unit V: Special Topics

The purpose of this unit is to provide descriptions and nursing implications for hemodynamic monitoring, administration of IV medications, administration of blood and blood products, and the delivery of home intravenous therapy. Chapter 13 describes the use of the subclavians, Swan-Ganz, and Hickman-Broviac catheters and arterial lines in hemodynamic monitoring. Chapter 14 includes a discussion of the types of incompatibility, factors affecting compatibility, and major nursing interventions for drug administration. Chapter 15 describes the types and administration of various blood products and includes a discussion of transfusion complications. Chapter 16 summarizes those clients qualifying for home IV therapy and specific implications for home administration.

Unit VI: Promoting Safety for the Intravenous Therapy Practitioner

The focus of this unit is promoting safety for the IV therapy practitioner. Chapter 17 describes an appreciation for the occupational hazards associated with working in IV therapy. Included are descriptions of both infectious and chemical hazards, suggested preventive measures, and treatment regimens. Chapter 18 discusses the quality assurance process, including standards of professional practice and product evaluation guidelines, legal implications of intravenous therapy, and the role of intravenous therapy teams.

References

NITA. 1986. The Importance of Intravenous Therapy. *Health Care Decisions*, (September) p 1.

Turco S. 1983. Clinical use of parenterals. *Parenterals* 1:4.

Acknowledgments

The authors wish to acknowledge their gratitude to those special friends, colleagues, and family members whose belief and support of this project enabled it to become a reality. Special thanks are extended to Diana Intenzo, Editor-in-Chief, Nursing Division, J. B. Lippincott Company, for her unwavering commitment to the development of this book; to Mary Murphy, Editorial Assistant, Nursing Division, for her continuous support and attention to detail; to Jody DeMatteo, Manuscript Editor, for her meticulousness in editing, patience, and sensitive, caring manner of relating; and to Donna Kubesh, M.S., R.N., and Jane Muhl, M.S., R.N., for reviewing the manuscript.

Contents

Unit I

Foundations of Intravenous Therapy

1 ▷ Principles and Assessment of Fluid and Electrolyte Balance

Key Points

1. Body fluid compartments
2. Water and electrolyte movement
3. Two basic rules of homeostatic fluid physiology
4. Achieving homeostasis
5. Major body fluid imbalances
6. Electrolytes
7. Acid–base balance
8. Patients at risk for fluid or electrolyte imbalance
9. Nursing observations related to body fluid imbalances
10. Useful laboratory values

Body Fluid Compartments

Approximately 60% of the total weight of the human body is composed of fluid, depending on age, sex, and body fat content. In general, infants, men, and leaner persons have higher percentages of body fluid. Approximately 45% of the body fluid is located inside of cells (intracellular) and 15% is located outside of cells (extracellular). Extracellular fluid can be further divided into 3% intravascular fluid (also known as the plasma, or liquid fraction of the blood) and 12% interstitial fluid (found outside the blood vessels in the interstitial spaces between body cells).

These three compartments, intracellular, intravascular, and interstitial, are separated from each other by membranes that allow water to pass. However, the membranes have different permeabilities to other substances. This means that the three compartments can each have different solutes dissolved in their water.

Body fluid consists mainly of various electrolytes dissolved in water, and its composition varies a great deal between body compartments. For example, intracellular fluid contains large amounts of potassium and phosphate, while plasma in the intravascular compartment contains much greater amounts of chloride and sodium. Body fluid compartments are separated by semipermeable membranes that allow both solute particles and fluids to move back and forth, depending on membrane pore size and the osmolality of the individual compartments. Osmolality is defined as a measure of the number of particles in a solution that reduces the concentration of body water and therefore changes its chemical behavior; osmolality is usually measured in milliosmoles per kilogram of fluid.

Water and Electrolyte Movement

Water and electrolytes move between the body fluid compartments in four basic ways: diffusion, osmosis, active transport, and filtration.

Diffusion

Diffusion is the random movement of molecules and ions from an area of higher concentration to an area of lower concentration. Ease and speed of diffusion of substances in and out of body fluids through semipermeable membranes depend on factors such as the following:

- Membrane permeability
- Size of the diffusing ion or molecule
- Differences in electrical potential
- Pressure gradients on either side of the membrane

Osmosis

Osmosis is the movement of water through a semipermeable membrane from an area where the water contains relatively few solute particles to an area of water that contains more solute particles.

1. Remember the phrase "water goes where the most solute particles are" when thinking about osmotic effect.
2. When no water movement occurs through a membrane owing to osmosis, the two solutions on either side of the membrane are said to be isotonic—each exerting the same amount of osmotic pressure because they each contain the same amount of osmotically active solute particles.
3. A fluid that contains a large number of solute particles would be hypertonic when compared with pure water containing no solute particles; pure water would be hypotonic when compared with a fluid containing many solute particles.

Active Transport

Active transport is a mechanism that involves the expenditure of cellular energy in the form of adenosine triphosphate (ATP) to move molecules through membranes against a concentration gradient.

Sodium–Potassium Pump

1. The sodium–potassium pump, an important example of active transport, is present in all cell membranes of the body. Both sodium and potassium ions can diffuse through cell membranes in small quantities. Their concentrations would eventually become equal inside and outside the cell over time, but the sodium–potassium pump, fueled by ATP, moves sodium back to the outside of the cell and potassium back to the inside of the cell against a concentration gradient.

2. The sodium–potassium pump is especially important in nerve and muscle fibers for transmission of impulses, in various glands for the secretion of different substances, and in all cells of the body to prevent cellular swelling. In a metabolically active cell, ATP fuels the pump to continually transport sodium to the exterior, taking excess water along with it to prevent the cell from swelling. Whenever the metabolism of the cell stops and ATP is no longer available to keep the pump working, the cell will immediately begin to swell and can eventually burst.

Filtration

Filtration is the movement of solutes and water through semipermeable membranes from an area of higher pressure to an area of lower pressure.

1. Dissolved substances and water are forced out of the arterial end of capillary beds through semipermeable membranes into the interstitial areas by the force of hydrostatic pressure created by the pumping action of the heart.
2. Filtration also occurs in the glomerular capillaries of the kidneys and forces water and electrolytes into the tubules.
3. The normal opposing force to capillary filtration is plasma colloid osmotic pressure. This tends to pull water from the interstitial area back into the intravascular compartment. This is accomplished by the magnetlike attraction that high-molecular-weight colloids found in the bloodstream (such as albumin and other proteins) have for water.
4. Any fluid not drawn back into the vascular compartment by plasma colloid osmotic pressure or returned to the vascular compartment by way of the lymphatic channels can accumulate in the interstitial space and cause edema (also known as third-space shifting). If plasma protein levels decrease, lymphatic channels become blocked, capillary permeability increases, or

capillary pressure increases, more fluid will leave the capillaries than will return, and edema will occur.

Two Basic Rules of Homeostatic Fluid Physiology

Homeostasis is thought of as being the normal state of relative constancy of the chemical and physical properties of body fluids. The human body follows two basic rules in achieving homeostasis within and between the body fluid compartments.

Rule 1

The overall amount and composition of fluid within each compartment must remain relatively stable, and within each compartment a state of electrical neutrality must exist.

1. While the basic composition and amount of fluid within each of the body compartments does stay the same, the compartments are constantly exchanging and replacing individual ions.
2. In addition, each fluid compartment must maintain electrical neutrality by balancing the number of cations and anions so that no net electrical charge occurs within the compartment.
3. Constantly controlling and maintaining this balance within each compartment can take up to 20% of the body's ATP energy stores.

Rule 2

The osmolality between the intracellular, interstitial, and intravascular fluid compartments must be equal. If the compartments differ in total number of osmotically active particles, water will tend to move into the compartment that contains the greater number of active particles. (See Major Body Fluid Imbalances, in this chapter.)

Achieving Homeostasis

Many organs of the body are associated with achieving, controlling, and maintaining the delicate balance of body fluids, electrolytes, and other compounds.

1. Kidneys
   - Often referred to as the "masters" of homeostasis because of the many critical functions they perform
   - Excrete chemical wastes and remove foreign substances from the blood that have been absorbed from the digestive tract
   - Produce bicarbonate and erythropoietin
   - Secrete renin
   - Convert one form of vitamin D into a more usable one
   - Control extracellular fluid by regulating electrolyte concentration, body fluid osmolality and volume, and blood pH and volume
2. Heart and blood vessels
   - Maintain blood flow to the kidneys
3. Lungs
   - Regulate oxygen and carbon dioxide levels in the blood
   - Allow water vapor to escape from the body
4. Skin
   - Allows perspiration and water vapor to escape from the body
5. Adrenal glands
   - Produce the mineralocorticoid hormone called aldosterone that acts on the kidney tubular cells and increases the reabsorption of sodium and water while decreasing potassium reabsorption
6. Hypothalamus
   - Contains osmoreceptors, which respond to increased body fluid osmolality and signal the sensation of thirst
   - Manufactures antidiuretic hormone (ADH, which is also called vasopressin); ADH causes kidney

tubular cells to reabsorb more water from the kidney filtrate; the body then retains more water and the urine becomes more concentrated
7. Pituitary gland
   - Stores and secretes ADH
8. Parathyroid glands
   - Control the level of ionized calcium in the blood by the secretion of parathyroid hormone
9. Gastrointestinal (GI) tract
   - Regulates water absorption and reabsorption

Major Body Fluid Imbalances

When the volume or composition of body fluid deviates even a small amount from normal, serious consequences can result. Which of the three fluid compartments of the body will be affected by either a gain or a loss of fluid will usually depend on the nature of that fluid and the rate at which it is gained or lost.

The intravascular compartment is considered to be the most accessible, since fluid is filtered from it by the kidneys, lungs, GI tract, and skin, and fluid can enter it from the GI tract. The intravascular compartment can also be accessed directly: intravenous (IV) fluids can be added to it, and fluid can be lost from it by hemorrhage. The intravascular compartment is affected the most by the gain or loss of a large amount of fluid over a short period.

Next in accessibility is the interstitial compartment, which functions almost like a storage area. If given a long enough time, the body can temporarily store excess fluid here, or fluid can be borrowed from this compartment if needed in another compartment.

The intracellular compartment is the least accessible of the three. It is protected from most fluid shifts by cellular membranes, except for those shifts brought about by osmotic pressure due to loss or gain of hypertonic or hypotonic solutions.

If a patient loses several liters of fluid in a few hours (*e.g.,* hemorrhage, massive diarrhea, or extensive burns), the loss will be borne mainly by the intravascular compartment, since a few hours is not enough time for the interstitial compartment to help replace the lost fluid. Shock will usually develop. Eventually, given enough time, the interstitial compartment can begin to move some of its fluid into the bloodstream to try to replace what was lost. If the fluid was lost over a longer period of time (such as over 24 hours), the interstitial compartment can be more efficient at replacing the lost fluid. When fluid is lost from the entire extracellular compartment (both intravascular and interstitial areas), a condition known as dehydration usually results.

Conversely, if a large amount of fluid is pumped into the intravascular compartment over a short period (*e.g.,* early postoperative patients receiving IV therapy), the fluid will not have a chance to move out into the interstitial compartment. Circulatory overload will probably result. If the fluid is gained over a longer period, some of the fluid will be able to be moved into the interstitial area for storage. When fluid is gained by the entire extracellular compartment, a condition known as peripheral edema usually results.

These previous examples of fluid loss or gain have described situations in which the fluid that was either lost or gained was isotonic fluid, meaning it contained the same number of solute particles as body fluid and consequently exerted no osmotic pressure. Losses or gains of isotonic fluid will not affect the intracellular fluid compartment, and the extracellular compartment will expand or contract in proportion to the amount of fluid gained or lost.

If the fluid lost from the body is hypotonic, such as pure water (*e.g.,* patients with increased insensible water loss), the rest of the extracellular fluid then becomes hypertonic and osmotically draws water away from the cells. This causes a fluid loss not only in the extracellular compartment but also in the intracellular compartment.

The opposite can occur if a hypotonic fluid such as pure water is added to the body (*e.g.,* patients receiving large amounts of electrolyte-free water to replace water lost from gastric suctioning): the hypotonic fluid will be drawn into all three fluid compartments because each contains a hypertonic solution. At that point, all three compartments, including the intracellular one, will have gained fluid. Changes in intracellular fluid that are caused by osmotic pressure often produce central nervous system (CNS) disturbances such as headache, nausea, confusion, disorientation, and convulsions.

In general, one should consider the type of fluid and the rate at which it was lost or gained, as well as which compartment the change will affect, when classifying body fluid disturbances. The patient who loses a lot of isotonic fluid very rapidly will develop shock (loss of extracellular fluid only). The patient who loses isotonic fluid slowly will usually not develop shock but will become dehydrated (again, loss of extracellular fluid only). The patient who loses pure water will become dehydrated and will probably exhibit some CNS symptoms but will probably not develop shock because the water loss will be shared by both the extracellular and the intracellular compartment.

Conversely, a patient could develop pulmonary edema or peripheral edema from the gain of isotonic fluid, depending on the rate of the gain (only extracellular gain). The patient who receives pure water will gain in both extracellular and intracellular compartments and will probably exhibit CNS disturbances.

Since fluid changes can occur quickly and bring about disastrous results, the nurse must constantly monitor the fluid status of any patient receiving IV therapy so that possible imbalances can be anticipated and recognized early. Tables 1-1 and 1-2 summarize the major body fluid imbalances, including a description of and the common reasons for each imbalance, signs and symptoms, and possible nursing interventions for caring for patients with these imbalances.

Electrolytes

The unit commonly used to measure electrolytes is the milliequivalent. This unit measures the chemical activity or chemical combining power of an ion. One milliequivalent of an anion will be able to combine chemically with 1 mEq of a cation, such as sodium (Na^+) combining with chloride (Cl^-). Laboratory values for electrolytes are usually expressed in milliequivalents per liter.

Functions

Electrolytes serve three major functions in homeostasis.

1. They influence body fluid osmolality and distribution.
2. They play an essential role in neuromuscular activity.
3. They help regulate acid–base balance to maintain normal pH.

Major Imbalances

Refer to Tables 1-3 to 1-10 for descriptions of the major imbalances that can occur with four important and commonly measured electrolytes (sodium, potassium, calcium, and magnesium). Also listed are the common reasons for each imbalance, signs and symptoms, and possible nursing interventions for caring for clients with these electrolyte imbalances. In addition, Tables 1-11 to 1-14 list possible changes in serum electrolyte levels that can be expected during each of the four major acid–base imbalances.

The reader is urged to consult the many fine articles and textbooks listed at the end of this chapter for a more in-depth look at the concepts of acid-base-electrolyte balance.

Acid–Base Balance

Acid–base balance involves a stable relationship between acids (molecules that give up hydrogen ions) and buffers (molecules that accept hydrogen ions). Since acids are by-products of cellular metabolism, they are being produced constantly by living cells and have a major affect on the acid–base balance in the body. Blood pH is determined by the amount of acid, or hydrogen ion, present. Normal pH of arterial blood is 7.40, with a normal range of between 7.35 and 7.45. Blood pH lower than 6.80 or higher than 7.80 is incompatible with human life. Therefore, the hydrogen ion concentration in the bloodstream must be carefully regulated by the body.

Normally, a ratio of 1 part acid to 20 parts buffer in the bloodstream keeps the pH within the normal range. Buffers are basically acid neutralizers: they combine with and render inactive the hydrogen ions given off by acid molecules and prevent them from altering the pH until they can be eliminated from the body.

Buffering Pathways

There are two main pathways for buffering and then eliminating acids from the body before the $1:20$ ratio of acid to buffer is upset.

1. Metabolic pathway
   - "Fixed acids" such as lactic, pyruvic, and acetoacetic, are formed during the incomplete breakdown of fats and sugars within cells; sulfuric and phosphoric fixed acids are produced as end products from the breakdown of proteins.
   - Fixed acids are buffered mainly by blood buffers such as bicarbonate, plasma proteins, and inorganic phosphates.
   - Fixed acids are eliminated from the body by the kidneys.
   - The metabolic pathway takes several days to speed up acid excretion in response to an increase in fixed acid production.
2. Respiratory pathway
   - This is a special pathway for the elimination of the large amount of carbon dioxide (CO_2) that is produced as a cellular waste product.

- CO_2 is sometimes called a volatile acid because if CO_2 gas comes into contact with water it may combine with it to produce carbonic acid, which will release hydrogen ions.
- Most of the CO_2 that is produced by cells remains dissolved in the bloodstream as CO_2 gas. The remainder that does form carbonic acid is buffered mainly by the hemoglobin contained in red blood cells, with help from organic phosphates and bicarbonate.
- Once in the lungs, buffered hydrogen ions are released from hemoglobin, carbonic acid is converted back into CO_2 and water, and the CO_2 is eliminated from the body in exchange for oxygen in the alveoli of the lung.

Acidosis/Alkalosis

If the 1:20 ratio of acid to buffer changes, one of two conditions can result.

1. *Acidosis* (increased amount of hydrogen ions in the bloodstream causing the pH to go below 7.35) may result when the body either gains acid or loses buffer, upsetting the normal 1:20 ratio. A large amount of acid can be produced during diabetic ketoacidosis, or buffer can be lost during diarrhea—both instances could eventually lead to acidosis.
2. *Alkalosis* (decreased amount of hydrogen ions in the bloodstream causing the pH to go above 7.45) may result when the body either loses acid or gains buffer, again upsetting the normal 1:20 ratio. Acid can be lost following prolonged vomiting, or buffer can be gained after ingestion of large amounts of bicarbonate of soda.

Metabolic and Respiratory Compensation

Because the metabolic and the respiratory components of the machinery for the handling of hydrogen ion are essentially independent of one another, one of the systems may compensate, to a certain extent, for a deficiency of the other system. This compensation may be partial or complete and is usually named for the system that is doing the compensating.

For example, during diabetic ketoacidosis, excess fixed acids produced in body cells are dumped into the bloodstream. The kidneys, whose job it is to remove these acids from the bloodstream and eliminate them from the body, will soon become overwhelmed by the extra acid load. Since it takes several days for the kidneys to speed up the rate of acid excretion in response to an extra acid load, many acids will have to remain in the bloodstream, causing a drop in pH that can result in metabolic acidosis. However, the respiratory system, which is much faster acting than the metabolic system, can help excrete some of these extra acids immediately. By causing the breathing rate to increase, extra CO_2 (which can be thought of as acid) will be blown off, the overall acid load will be decreased, and the pH should remain within normal limits, at least for a while. Diabetic patients who are in ketoacidosis frequently exhibit a type of rapid, deep breathing known as Kussmaul's respiration in an attempt to rid the body of extra acid. This is an example of the respiratory compensation mechanism.

Major Acid–Base Disturbances

Tables 1-11 to 1-14 describe the major acid–base imbalances that can occur, including common reasons for each imbalance, compensation mechanisms that may occur, signs and symptoms of the imbalance, and possible nursing interventions.

The reader is urged to consult the many fine articles and textbooks listed at the end of this chapter for a more in-depth look at the concepts of acid-base-electrolyte balance.

Patients at Risk for Fluid or Electrolyte Imbalance

During an average day the human body processes approximately 2½ quarts of liquid and approximately 2⅓ g (100 mEq) of sodium, plus a few other electrolytes and related compounds. It is the responsibility of the organs of homeostasis to control how much water, along with which electrolytes and in what specific amounts, will be kept in the body and which will be excreted to maintain homeostasis. It is the responsibility of the nurse to anticipate and recognize possible problems with homeostatic mechanisms that patients may encounter.

Certain patients, owing to underlying disease or medical treatment, will be at greater risk for developing a fluid or electrolyte disturbance than others. It is important that these patients be identified early and monitored closely for any evidence of abnormalities. Any of the following can serve as a clue to possible impending fluid or electrolyte problems: very young or very old patients; disease states such as diabetes, congestive heart failure, alcoholism, adrenal insufficiency, pancreatitis, peritonitis, meningitis, pneumonia, thyroid imbalance, and renal insufficiency or failure; conditions such as fever, diarrhea, vomiting, excessive sweating, excessive wound drainage, burns, crushing injuries, and head injuries; ingestion or administration of drugs such as steroids, diuretics, potassium compounds, barbiturates, salicylates, hormones, blood and blood products, and certain over-the-counter medications such as antacids or cathartics; treatment procedures such as mechanical ventilation, gastric suctioning, anesthesia, any type of surgery (especially abdominal surgery), parenteral administration of solutions, prolonged immobilization, tight dressings, diet restrictions, and fluid restrictions.

The list goes on and on, but the main idea is that almost every patient hospitalized today will be at some risk of developing a fluid or electrolyte imbalance. Early recognition of the predisposing factors will allow for plan-

(*Text continues on p. 48*)

Table 1-1. Fluid Volume Excess

Type and Description	Common Reasons for the Imbalance
Circulatory overload (gain of isotonic fluid that causes the ECF volume to increase)	Administration of isotonic IV solutions, especially to early post-op, post trauma, elderly, or stressed patients
Water intoxication (gain of hypotonic fluid that causes both ECF and ICF volumes to increase)	Administration of large quantities of electrolyte-free water to replace fluid and electrolytes lost from gastric suction, vomiting, diarrhea, diuresis, or perspiration Administration of 5% dextrose in water (sugar is quickly metabolized in the bloodstream, leaving the hypotonic water) Administration of IV fluids to early postop, stressed, or elderly patients or patients with impaired renal function

Signs and Symptoms	Nursing Interventions
Weight gain	Assess
Positive fluid balance	Vital signs
High pulse pressure, bounding and not easily obliterated	I and O
Daily weight	
Increased central venous pressure	Neck vein distention and presence of pulmonary edema
Peripheral edema	Lab values
Slow-emptying hand veins when arm is raised	Restrict fluids as ordered by physician
Cyanosis	Administer diuretics as ordered by physician
Dyspnea	
Coughing	Reduce pressure on skin areas
Jugular vein distention	
Pulmonary edema	
Lab values show drop in hematocrit, hemoglobin, and total protein	
Weight gain	Assess
Positive fluid balance	Vital signs
Blood pressure usually normal but may be elevated	I and O
Daily weight	
Nerve function	
Pulse may be regular and not easily obliterated	Behavior
Lab values	
Slow-emptying hand veins when arm is raised	Restrict fluids as ordered by physician
Acute onset of behavioral changes: disorientation, confusion, apathy, irritability	Administer small amounts of 3% or 5% NaCl in water as ordered by physician
CNS disturbances: headaches, nausea, vomiting, weakness, muscle twitching, convulsions	
Lab values show drop in hematocrit, hemoglobin, total protein, and serum sodium	

Continued

Table 1-1. (Continued)

Type and Description	Common Reasons for the Imbalance
Hypertonic expansion (gain of hypertonic fluid that causes ECF volume to increase and ICF volume to decrease; water is drawn from the ICF to the ECF owing to osmotic pressure)	IV administration of hypertonic solutions (usually saline) intended to replace massive sodium loss or to remove excess accumulation of body fluids

(*ECF,* extracellular fluid; *ICF,* intracellular fluid; *I and O,* intake and output)

Signs and Symptoms	Nursing Interventions

Weight gain, depending on amount infused	Assess
	   Vital signs
	   I and O
	   Daily weight
	   Neck vein distention and presence of peripheral edema
	   Behavior
	   Lab values

Intense thirst (may be absent in elderly)	
Full, bounding pulse	
In early stages, peripheral edema, diminished skin turgor	
Slow-emptying hand veins when arm is raised	Restrict fluids as ordered by physician
In late stages, pulmonary edema	Administer 5% dextrose in water as ordered by physician
Restlessness, excitement, agitation	Reduce pressure on skin areas
Lab values show drop in hematocrit, hemoglobin, and total protein; serum sodium is increased	

Table 1-2. Fluid Volume Deficit

Type and Description	Common Reasons for the Imbalance
Hypovolemia (loss of isotonic fluid that causes the ECF volume to decrease)	Loss of whole blood Loss of large volume of fluid from diarrhea, vomiting, fistulous drainage Systemic infections causing fever and increased utilization of water and electrolytes
Hypotonic dehydration (loss of fluids containing relatively more salt than water, causing ECF volume to decrease and ICF volume to increase; water is drawn from the ECF to the ICF owing to osmotic pressure)	Urine loss in patients receiving diuretics Fistula drainage Severe burns Perspiration Vomitus Elderly patients especially affected by loss of small amounts of sodium

(*ECF*, extracellular fluid; *ICF*, intracellular fluid; *I and O*, intake and output)

Signs and Symptoms	Nursing Interventions
Weight loss	Assess
Negative fluid balance	Vital signs
Regular pulse rate but easily obliterated	I and O
	Daily weight
Decreased central venous pressure	Skin turgor
	Lab values
Slow-filling hand veins when arm is lowered	Replace lost fluids with isotonic IV solutions as ordered by physician
Flat neck veins in supine position	
Pinched facial expression	
Decreased skin turgor (in youth and the middle-aged)	
Decreased tearing and salivation	
Lab values show increase in hematocrit, hemoglobin, and total protein	
Weight loss	Assess
Negative fluid balance	Vital signs
Pulse rate increased, easily obliterated, and weak or thready	I and O
	Daily weight
	Skin turgor
Slow-filling hand veins when arm is lowered	Nerve function
	Behavior
Decreased skin turgor (in youth and the middle-aged)	Lab values
CNS disturbances: headache, nausea, cramps, vomiting	Replace the lost fluids and electrolytes, usually with balanced electrolyte IV solutions, as ordered by physician
Behavioral changes: apathy and confusion	
Lab values show increase in hematocrit, hemoglobin, and total protein; serum sodium is decreased	

Continued

Table 1-2. (Continued)

Type and Description	Common Reasons for the Imbalance
Hypertonic dehydration (loss of water without a corresponding loss of salt, causing both ECF and ICF volumes to decrease)	Patients unable to take in sufficient fluid over a long period
	Excess insensible water loss through lungs or skin
	Tracheobronchitis
	Frequently seen in elderly because of decreased thirst stimulus

(*ECF*, extracellular fluid; *ICF*, intracellular fluid; *I and O*, intake and output)

Signs and Symptoms	**Nursing Interventions**
Weight loss	Assess
Negative fluid balance	Vital signs
Thirst (may be absent in the elderly)	I and O
	Daily weight
Pulse normal and regular in early stages	Mucous membranes
	Skin turgor
Hand vein filling time usually normal in early stages	Thirst
	Nerve function
Dry, sticky mucous membranes	Behavior
	Lab values
Dry mouth with furrowed tongue	In early stages administer plain water by mouth as ordered by physician
Skin turgor diminishes as condition progresses	In more advanced stages rehydrate client, administer balanced hypotonic IV solutions as ordered by physician
Patient may have fever	
Restlessness, irritability, and confusion	
Decreased reflexes, may develop mania or convulsions	Administer potassium-sparing diuretics as ordered by physician
Lab values show increase in hematocrit, hemoglobin, total protein, and serum sodium	

Table 1-3. Hypernatremia

Description of Imbalance	Common Reasons for the Imbalance

Serum sodium above 145 mEq/liter	Conditions of increased water loss:
	     Diabetes insipidus
	     Osmotic diuresis
	     Renal concentrating disorders
	     Prolonged diarrhea
	     Excessive sweating
	
	 Conditions of decreased water intake or increased salt intake:
	     No thirst response
	     No access to water
	     Difficulty in swallowing
	     High solute intake (tube feedings)
	     Administration of hypertonic NaCl
	     Hyperaldosteronism
	     Cushing's syndrome

Signs and Symptoms	Nursing Interventions
Extreme thirst	Assess
Tongue rough, red, and dry	Vital signs
Skin flushed	Intake and output
Temperature elevated	Daily weight
Restlessness	Skin turgor and color
Excitement	Mucous membranes
Agitation	Nerve function
Confusion	Behavior
	Lab values
Muscle weakness and twitching	Monitor replacement of lost water as ordered by physician
Oliguria or anuria	Give water between tube feedings
Convulsions	
Coma	Use humidified air during mechanical ventilation and check water level regularly

Lab values:
  Serum sodium above 145 mEq/liter
  Urine specific gravity above 1.030
	Encourage decreased sodium food intake

	Give low-sodium foods orally
	Refrain from giving saline laxatives
	Refrain from giving table salt
	Substitute artificial salt
	Explain the causes of the problem
	Explain the reason for and intended effect of therapy
	Instruct patients to drink 8 to 10 glasses of water daily
	Teach elderly to drink water daily
	Teach patients which foods contain large amounts of sodium

Table 1-4. Hyponatremia

Description of Imbalance	Common Reasons for the Imbalance
Serum sodium below 135 mEq/liter	Conditions of increased water intake (water intoxication): Excessive tap-water enemas Stimulation of ADH Adrenal insufficiency Psychogenic polydipsia Conditions of increased salt loss: Use of hypotonic irrigation solutions Diuretic therapy Replacement of water but not electrolytes lost in burns, sweating, vomiting, diarrhea, and nasogastric suctioning

Signs and Symptoms	Nursing Interventions
Malaise	Assess
Headache	Vital signs
Confusion	Intake and output
Lethargy	Daily weight
Dizziness	Nerve function
Postural hypotension	Behavior
Personality change	GI function
	Lab values
Cold and clammy skin	Help patients comply with fluid restrictions as ordered by physician
Abdominal cramps, nausea, vomiting, diarrhea	
Apprehension	Use normal saline for irrigations
Convulsions	Give isotonic ice chips to patients receiving nasogastric suctioning
Coma	
Lab values:	Avoid tap-water enemas
Serum sodium below 135 mEq/liter	Explain the causes of the problem
Urine specific gravity below 1.010	Explain the reason for and intended effect of therapy
	Teach patients to replace lost fluid with juice or bouillon instead of water

Table 1-5. Hyperkalemia

Description of Imbalance	Common Reasons for the Imbalance
Serum potassium above 5 mEq/liter	Condition of increased K^+ intake: 　Excess or too rapid IV administration Conditions of decreased urinary excretion of K^+: 　Renal failure 　K^+-sparing diuretics 　Decreased effect of aldosterone Movement of K^+ into extracellular fluid: 　Acidosis 　Insulin deficiency 　Tissue injury 　Massive digitalis overdose

Signs and Symptoms	Nursing Interventions
Irritability	Assess
Nausea	Vital signs
Diarrhea	Muscle strength
Intestinal colic	Behavior
Muscle weakness	GI function
Flaccid paralysis	Lab values
Oliguria, may progress to anuria	Increase fluids as ordered to increase urinary output
Cardiac arrhythmias	Provide adequate nutrition to prevent tissue breakdown
Cardiac arrest	If physician orders cation exchange resin, monitor for constipation
Lab values:	Withhold foods and drugs with high K^+ content
Serum potassium above 5 mEq/liter	Explain the causes of the problem
Hyperkalemia often accompanies metabolic acidosis	Explain the reason for and intended effect of therapy
	Teach patients about the use of K^+-sparing diuretics
	Teach patients to recognize signs of hyperkalemia

Table 1-6. Hypokalemia

Description of Imbalance	Common Reasons for the Imbalance

Serum potassium below 3.5 mEq/liter	Condition of decreased K^+ intake:
	    Anorexia
	
	Conditions of K^+ loss:
	    Vomiting
	    Bulemia
	    Nasogastric suction
	    Diarrhea
	    Laxative abuse
	    Large sweat loss without replacement
	    Increased urinary secretion from increased effect of aldosterone
	    Diuretics
	    Renal salt wasting
	    Hypomagnesemia
	
	Movement of K^+ from extracellular fluid into cells:
	    Alkalosis
	    Hypersecretion of insulin

Signs and Symptoms	Nursing Interventions
Malaise	Assess
Polyuria	Vital signs
Thirst	Muscle strength
Muscle weakness	Behavior
Flaccid paralysis	Possible digitalis toxicity
Cardiac disturbances	Lab values
Anorexia	Administer IV K^+ (or NaCl if alkalosis is present) slowly as ordered by physician
Nausea	
Vomiting	If K^+ is given orally, watch for GI irritation
Intestinal distention	
Paralytic ileus	Explain the causes of the problem
Weakness of respiratory muscles—shallow respiration	Explain the reason for and intended effect of therapy
Respiratory arrest	Teach patients which foods contain high K^+ content
Lab values:	
Serum potassium below 3.5 mEq/liter	Teach patients about use of K^+ supplements
Hypokalemia often accompanies metabolic alkalosis	Teach patients about use of diuretics

Table 1-7.   Hypercalcemia

Description of Imbalance	Common Reasons for the Imbalance

Serum calcium above 11 mg/dl	Conditions of increased GI absorption:
	   Hypervitaminosis D
	   Milk–alkali syndrome
	   Sarcoidosis
	
	Conditions of increased calcium release from bone:
	   Malignancy
	   Hyperparathyroidism
	   Bone tumors
	   Multiple myeloma
	   Leukemia
	   Prolonged immobilization
	
	Increase in physiologically available calcium:
	   Acidosis

Signs and Symptoms	Nursing Interventions
Muscle weakness	Assess
Deep bony pain	Vital signs
Pathologic fractures	Muscle strength
Headache	Bone or flank pain
Fatigue	Behavior
Confusion	GI function
Lethargy	Possible digitalis toxicity
CNS depression	Lab values
Anorexia	Administer IV NaCl as ordered by physician
Vomiting	Administer diuretics as ordered by physician
Nausea	Administer phosphates, glucocorticoids, or calcitonin as ordered by physician
Abdominal pain	Ensure adequate hydration
Constipation	Maintain an acid urine
Dehydration	Handle patient gently when moving or turning
Flank pain	Increase patient mobility
Renal calculi	Explain the causes of the problem
Polyuria	Explain the reason for and intended effect of therapy
Azotemia	Teach patients to avoid excess vitamin D supplements and over-the-counter medicines containing calcium
Renal failure	Teach patients the importance of mobility and exercise as tolerated
Stupor	
Coma	
Cardiac arrest	
Lab values:	
Serum calcium above 11 mg/dl	
Elevated BUN if stones have damaged kidneys	
Hypercalcemia often accompanies metabolic acidosis	

Table 1-8. Hypocalcemia

Description of Imbalance	Common Reasons for the Imbalance
Serum calcium below 8.5 mg/dl	Conditions of decreased intake or GI absorption: Sprue Steatorrhea Diarrhea Overuse of antacids Long-term use of laxatives Pancreatitis Dietary lack of milk or vitamin D Chronic uremia Conditions of increased calcium loss or excretion: Chronic renal insufficiency Use of diuretics Burns Peritonitis Decrease in physiologically available calcium: Alkalosis Massive blood transfusion Hypoparathyroidism Overuse of phosphate-containing laxatives Surgical removal or damage to the parathyroid glands

Signs and Symptoms	**Nursing Interventions**
Tingling in ends of fingers and perioral area	Assess
Muscle twitching and cramping	Vital signs
Carpopedal spasms	Neuromuscular function
Tetany	GI function
Laryngeal stridor	Presence of positive Chvostek's sign and Trousseau's sign (see page 50)
Convulsions	Lab values
Bone fractures (in chronic hypocalcemia)	Administer vitamin D, magnesium, or calcium as ordered by physician
Lab values:	Keep 10% calcium gluconate available for emergency IV administration to treat tetany or convulsions as ordered by physician
Serum calcium below 8.5 mg/dl	Encourage patient mobility
Hypocalcemia often accompanies metabolic alkalosis	Explain the causes of the problem
	Explain the reason for and intended effect of therapy
	Teach patients careful antacid and laxative management
	Teach adults the importance of consuming dairy products as tolerated
	Teach patients that tetany can be exacerbated by hyperventilation or pressure on efferent nerves (*e.g.*, crossing legs)
	Teach patients the importance of mobility and exercise as tolerated

Table 1-9. Hypermagnesemia

Description of Imbalance	Common Reasons for the Imbalance
Serum magnesium above 2.1 mEq/liter	Conditions of increased intake:
Neuromuscular excitability is decreased	Overuse of magnesium-containing cathartics
	Overuse of magnesium during replacement therapy
	Conditions of impaired excretion:
	Chronic renal failure
	Adrenal insufficiency

Signs and Symptoms	Nursing Interventions
CNS depression	Assess
Lethargy	Vital signs
Drowsiness	Neuromuscular function
Hypotension	Behavior
Sweating	Lab values
Flushing	Give fluids to increase urinary output as ordered by physician
Slow and weak pulse	
Weak or absent deep tendon reflexes	Withhold preparations containing magnesium
Flaccid paralysis	Keep 10% calcium gluconate available for emergency IV administration as ordered by physician
Respiratory depression	
Cardiac arrhythmias	
Cardiac arrest	
Lab values:	Explain the causes of the problem
Serum magnesium above 2.1 mEq/liter	
	Explain the reason for and intended effect of therapy
	Teach patients careful management of antacids and cathartics
	Teach patients having renal problems to avoid preparations that contain magnesium

Table 1-10. Hypomagnesemia

Description of Imbalance	Common Reasons for the Imbalance
Serum magnesium below 1.5 mEq/liter	Conditions of decreased intake or absorption:
	Chronic malnutrition
	Chronic diarrhea
	Malabsorption syndrome
	Bowel resection
	Chronic alcoholism
Neuromuscular excitability is increased	Conditions of gastrointestinal loss:
	Prolonged nasogastric suction
	Steatorrhea
	Acute pancreatitis
	Biliary or intestinal fistula
	Conditions of increased urinary excretion:
	Diuretic therapy
	Diabetic ketoacidosis
	Primary aldosteronism
	Renal reabsorption defect

Signs and Symptoms	Nursing Interventions
Insomnia	Assess
Confusion	Vital signs
Tremor	Neuromuscular function
Leg or foot cramps	Behavior
Hyperactive reflexes	Presence of positive
Carpopedal spasms	Chvostek's sign and Trous-
Tetany	seau's sign (see page 50)
Tachycardia	Lab values
Hallucinations	Check renal function before
Convulsions	administration of magnesium
Lab values:	Administer oral, intramuscu-
Serum magnesium below	lar, or intravenous magne-
1.5 mEq/liter	sium salts as ordered by
	physician
	Administer IV magnesium
	slowly to prevent patients
	from feeling flushed or hot
	Explain the causes of the
	problem
	Explain the reason for and
	intended effect of therapy
	Provide diet counseling for
	patients at risk

Table 1-11. Metabolic Acidosis

Description of Imbalance	Common Reasons for the Imbalance	Compensation Mechanism
Low pH Low HCO_3^- Pco_2 normal (until lungs compensate)	Addition of excess H^+ Diabetic ketoacidosis Renal failure Lactic acidosis (cardiac arrest, shock, hypoxia) Loss of HCO_3^- Diarrhea	Lungs will try to reduce Pco_2 by hyperventilation (possible Kussmaul's breathing); lungs can compensate quickly

Signs and Symptoms	Nursing Interventions

CNS depression
  Headache
  Fatigue
  Drowsiness
	Assess
	  Vital signs
	  Hourly intake and output
	  Daily weight

Decreased mental function: confusion and eventually coma	Skin color and temperature
	  Nerve function
	  GI function

Hypotension	Muscle strength Signs and symptoms of
Kussmaul's breathing	hyperkalemia
Tissue hypoxia	Lab values
Anorexia, nausea, and vomiting	Administer fluids and medicines as ordered by physician
Cardiac arrhythmia	Institute seizure precautions
Seizures	Maintain bed rest

Lab values:
  Serum sodium
    May be normal; total sodium is low if diuresis occurs
	Provide range-of-motion exercises
	
	Provide frequent oral hygiene

Serum potassium Will be high, although there will be overall cellular depletion of K^+	Maintain orientation to person, time, and place Provide comfort measures
Serum chloride May increase to replace lost HCO_3^-; if anion gap increases, Cl^- may decrease or be normal	
Urine pH Very low, as kidneys try to excrete H^+	

Table 1-12. Metabolic Alkalosis

Description of Imbalance	Common Reasons for the Imbalance	Compensation Mechanism
High HCO_3^- High pH Pco_2 normal (until lungs compensate)	Excess ingestion or infusion of HCO_3^- Vomiting or gastric suctioning, causing loss of H^+, Cl^-, and K^+ Renal loss from aldosterone excess Diuretic use leading to loss of H^+ and K^+	Lungs will try to increase Pco_2 slightly by hypoventilation (can be done quickly)

Signs and Symptoms	Nursing Interventions

CNS stimulation
  Confusion
  Irritability
  Belligerence
  Disorientation
Muscle weakness and cramps
Carpopedal spasms
Tetany
Polyuria
Polydipsia
Nausea, vomiting, and diarrhea
Hypoventilation
Seizures
Stupor
Coma
 	
Lab values:
  Serum sodium
    Usually not changed
  Serum potassium
    Low
  Serum chloride
    Low
  Urine pH
    High or paradoxically low owing to low amounts of K^+ and Cl^- present in kidney filtrate for reabsorption exchange of Na^+—this is known as "paradoxical aciduria"
	Assess
	  Vital signs
	  Intake and output
	  Daily weight
	  Level of consciousness
	  Neuromuscular function
	  Muscle strength
	  Patient comfort level
	  Presence of positive Chvostek's sign and Trousseau's sign (see page 50)
	  Lab values
	
	Administer fluids and meds as ordered by physician
	Establish a safe physical environment, including use of padded side rails
	Institute seizure precautions
	Maintain orientation to person, time, and place
	Provide emotional support and reassurance

Table 1-13. Respiratory Acidosis

Description of Imbalance	Common Reasons for the Imbalance	Compensation Mechanism

High Pco_2
Low pH
HCO_3^- normal (until kidneys compensate)
	Hypoventilation related to mechanical activity of respiratory system; causes include:
	  COPD
	  Emphysema
	  Asthma
	  Bronchitis
	  Polio
	  Spinal cord trauma
	  Pneumonia
	  Guillain-Barré syndrome
	
	Depression of respiratory centers due to:
	  Drug overdose
	  Barbiturate toxicity
	  Alcohol ingestion
	  Oversedation
	  General anesthesia
	  Head trauma
	  Central sleep apnea
		Kidneys will eventually retain more HCO_3^- (takes several days to complete)

Signs and Symptoms	Nursing Interventions

CNS depression
  Headache
  Fatigue
  Drowsiness
Decreased mental function
  Confusion
  Disorientation
  Coma
	Assess
	  Vital signs
	  Level of consciousness
	  Skin color, temperature,
	  and moistness
	  Muscle strength
	  Patient comfort level
	  Lab values

Fatigue and weakness	Decrease anxiety
Decreased reflexes, tremors, uncoordination	Minimize activity
Hypoventilation	Assist with activities of daily living
Dyspnea	Maintain orientation to person, time, and place
Tachycardia or other cardiac arrhythmia	Position for optimum respiratory function
Cyanosis	Assist with turning, coughing, and deep breathing

Lab values:
  Serum sodium
    Not usually changed
  Serum potassium
    May be slightly increased
  Serum chloride
    During compensation an increase in HCO_3^- will cause a decrease in Cl^-
  Urine pH
    Low, as many H^+ are being excreted by the kidneys
	Administer oxygen as ordered by physician
	Administer fluids and medicines as ordered by physician
	Provide emotional support
	Have emergency equipment ready

Table 1-14. Respiratory Alkalosis

Description of Imbalance	Common Reasons for the Imbalance	Compensation Mechanism
Low Pco_2 High pH HCO_3^- normal (until kidneys compensate)	Psychogenic Anxiety Pain Toxic stimulation of the respiratory center High fever, shock, bacteremia CNS disturbances (pulmonary embolism, excessive artificial respiration, interstitial lung disease) Drugs (salicylates, epinephrine)	Kidneys will eventually reduce the HCO_3^- (takes several days to complete)

Signs and Symptoms	**Nursing Interventions**

CNS stimulation
  Irritability
  Light-headed
  Ringing in ears
	Assess
	  Vital signs
	  Level of consciousness
	  Sensation in face and
	  extremities

Dizziness	Muscle strength
Sweating	Patient comfort level
Tingling in fingers and toes	Presence of positive
Numbness of extremities and perioral area	Chvostek's sign and Trous- seau's sign (see page 50)
Anxiety	Lab values
Cramps	Administer fluids and medicines as ordered by
Carpopedal spasms	physician
Altered consciousness	Establish a safe physical
Hypotension	environment, including use
Cardiac arrhythmias	of padded side rails
Seizures	Institute seizure precau- tions

Lab values:
  Serum sodium
    Usually not changed
  Serum potassium
    May be low if alkalinity
    persists
	Maintain orientation to
	person, time, and place
	
	Assist with turning, cough-
	ing, and deep breathing

Serum chloride
    Will be increased when
    HCO_3^- decreases during
    compensation phase
  Urine pH
    Will be high if respira-
    tory alkalosis is a
    chronic problem
	Provide emotional support
	and reassurance

ning, monitoring, and detection of the imbalance followed by early control or treatment.

Nursing Observations Related to Body Fluid Imbalances

General nursing observations and procedures can become valuable tools for recognizing and evaluating fluid or electrolyte problems:

1. *Body temperature.*
    - Fever can cause an increase in metabolic rate that results in extra waste products being produced that can be excreted only when dissolved in extra body fluid.
    - Fever also increases the respiratory rate and results in loss of more fluid through water vapor.
    - Elevated body temperature can indicate a sodium excess.
    - Lowered body temperature can indicate a fluid volume deficit.
2. *Pulse.* Pulse should be evaluated according to rate, volume, irregularity, and ease of obliteration. Pulse variations and their possible significance include the following:
    - Increased rate can mean: sodium excess, magnesium deficit, or hypovolemia
    - Decreased rate can mean: magnesium excess
    - Weak, irregular, and rapid can mean: severe potassium deficit
    - Weak, irregular, and slow can mean: severe potassium excess
    - Bounding and not easily obliterated can mean: circulatory overload or fluid volume excess
    - Bounding and easily obliterated can mean: impending circulatory collapse
    - Rapid, weak, and thready can mean: hypovolemia and impending circulatory collapse
    - Normal pulse suggests: a normal fluid balance

3. *Respirations*. Respirations should be evaluated according to rate, depth, and regularity.
   - Metabolic acidosis causes an increase in rate and depth.
   - Metabolic alkalosis causes a decrease in rate and depth.
4. *Blood pressure*.
   - Hypertension can signal magnesium deficit or hypervolemia.
   - Hypotension can mean magnesium excess or potassium deficit.
5. *Skin and mucous membranes*.
   - Dry mucous membranes and poor skin turgor usually indicate fluid volume deficit.
   - Dry, sticky mucous membranes are sometimes seen with hypernatremia (excess of serum sodium).
   - Cold, clammy, pale skin suggests decreased plasma volume.
   - Pitting edema indicates fluid volume excess.
6. *Hand and neck veins*. Normally, elevated hand veins empty in 3 to 5 seconds and lowered hand veins refill in 3 to 5 seconds. This guideline may not apply in elderly patients, who may have sclerosed or fragile veins.
   - Hypovolemia will cause the hand veins to appear less visible than usual and take longer than 5 seconds to fill.
   - Hypervolemia will cause the hand veins to appear engorged and take longer than 5 seconds to empty.
   - Distended neck veins can mean that the heart is unable to adequately receive and pump venous blood, which is an indication of increased central venous pressure.
7. *Behavior*. Changes in personality and activity level can be brought about by disturbances in pH, fluid level, or electrolyte balance.
   - Acidosis causes CNS depression, while alkalosis causes CNS stimulation.

- Depression and indifference can indicate hypervolemia.
- Irritability and restlessness can mean sodium or potassium excess.
- Speech pattern changes may point to fluid, potassium, or calcium imbalances.
- Muscle weakness and overall fatigue usually indicate a potassium imbalance, most often hypokalemia.
- Positive Chvostek's sign (patient's upper lip twitches when the facial nerve adjacent to the ear is tapped) and positive Trousseau's sign (carpopedal spasm that occurs spontaneously or after circulation to the hand is constricted by application of a blood pressure cuff) can mean calcium deficit, magnesium deficit, or alkalosis (ionization of calcium is decreased in an alkaline medium).
- Flaccid paralysis of the extremities and the respiratory muscles can occur with severe potassium excess or deficit.

8. *Thirst*. Thirst may indicate a deficit of body fluid, but this is not always the case.
   - The elderly patient often has a decreased thirst sensation and can become dehydrated before the condition is discovered.
   - Severely burned patients may experience great thirst; if they ingest excess water it can lead to serious sodium deficit.

9. *Weight*. One of the best indicators of fluid status is the patient's daily weight.
   - A loss of weight will be seen when total fluid intake is less than total fluid output, and weight gain will occur when intake is greater than output.
   - It is important to weigh the patient at the same time every day, use the same scale, and have the patient wear the same amount of clothing.
   - Remember: Daily weight does *not* reflect third-space shifting.

Table 1-15. Approximate Electrolyte Content (mEq/liter) of Selected Body Fluids and Possible Imbalance(s) Following Fluid Loss

Body Fluid	Na$^+$	K$^+$	Cl$^-$	Imbalance Following Loss
Gastric	60	10	100	Metabolic alkalosis; sodium, potassium, magnesium deficits; tetany; ketosis of starvation
Bile	140	10	100	Metabolic acidosis; sodium deficit
Intestinal	50	10	60	Extracellular fluid volume deficit; metabolic acidosis; sodium and potassium deficits
Pancreatic	140	10	75	Metabolic acidosis; decrease in extracellular fluid volume; sodium and calcium deficits
Perspiration	50	5	60	Sodium deficit (following ingestion of plain water); sodium excess (inadequate water intake)

(Adapted from Metheny N, Snively WD: *Nurse's Handbook of Fluid Balance,* 4th ed. Philadelphia, JB Lippincott, 1983.)

10. *Intake and output records.* Accurate intake and output records (I and O) can provide valuable information about fluid balance if done correctly.
    - Patients with the following conditions should automatically have I and O measurements recorded: following surgery (especially abdominal or bowel), renal failure, congestive heart failure, coma, diuretic therapy, known fluid or electrolyte imbalance, abnormal loss of body fluids, severe injury, trauma, or burns.
    - Every effort should be made to record I and O as accurately and as carefully as possible.

Table 1-16. Laboratory Values Useful in Evaluating Fluid Status

Laboratory Test Reference Value		Implication
Hematocrit Measures percentage by volume of packed red blood cells in whole blood	Adult female: 38% to 47% Adult male: 40% to 54%	Increases with dehydration Decreases with low red blood cell count Decreases with water overload
Blood Urea Nitrogen Reflects protein intake and renal excretory capacity	8–23 mg/dl	Increases with dehydration Decreases with water overload
Creatinine (serum) Measures glomerular filtration rate	0.6–1.5 mg/dl	Increases when renal disease damages 50% or more of nephrons
Osmolality (serum) Measures number of particles dissolved in body water that exert osmotic pull	280–295 mOsm/kg	Increases with dehydration Decreases with water overload
Specific Gravity (urine) Measures kidneys' ability to concentrate urine	1.016–1.022 (normal fluid intake) 1.001–1.035 (range)	Increases with dehydration Decreases with diabetes insipidus or acute renal failure, or when tubules lose the ability to concentrate urine

- Common errors include failure to estimate perspiration, wound exudate, lost irrigation fluid, vomitus, and liquid feces; failure to communicate I and O needs and rules to patient, family, and staff.

11. *Assessing the loss of specific body fluids.* The type of imbalance that occurs following the loss of a specific body fluid varies with the content of the lost fluid. Table 1-15 lists the major body fluids, their approximate electrolyte content, and the imbalance(s) that can result following the loss of certain fluids.

Useful Laboratory Values

No single magic laboratory or diagnostic test exists that will solely and accurately describe a patient's fluid status. The best that one can do is to look at a wide variety of parameters and try to piece together all the clues and information available into a composite picture of the fluid situation. Table 1-16 lists several laboratory tests that are helpful in evaluating fluid status when used along with other clinical parameters.

Bibliography

Arieff A, DeFronzo R (eds): Fluid, Electrolyte, and Acid-Base Disorders, vol. 1. New York, Churchill Livingstone, 1985

Folk-Lighty M: Solving the puzzles of patients' fluid imbalances. Nursing84 14:34, 1984

Glass LB, Jenkins CA: The ups and downs of serum pH. Nursing83, 13:34, 1983

Goldberger E: A Primer of Water, Electrolyte, and Acid-Base Syndromes, 6th ed. Philadelphia, Lea & Febiger, 1980

Guyton AC: Textbook of Medical Physiology, 6th ed. Philadelphia, WB Saunders, 1981

Kenner C, Dossey B (eds): Critical Care Nursing: Body, Mind, and Spirit, 2nd ed. Boston, Little, Brown & Co, 1985

Mandell HN: Gases and 'lytes without anguish. Postgrad Med 69:67, 1981

Metheny NM, Snively WD: Nurses' Handbook of Fluid Balance, 4th ed. Philadelphia, JB Lippincott, 1983

Miller W: The ABC's of blood gases. Emergency Med 16:36, 1984

Nursing Skillbook: Monitoring Fluid and Electrolytes Precisely. Springhouse, PA, Intermed Communications, 1983

Rice V: Problems of water regulation: Diabetes insipidus and syndromes of inappropriate antidiuretic hormone. Crit Care Nurse 3:63, 1983

Romanski S: Interpreting ABG's in four easy steps. Nursing86, 16:58, 1986

Stark J: Water regulation in health and renal disease. NITA 8:497, 1985

Stroot VR, Lee CA, Barrett CA: Fluids and Electrolytes: A Practical Approach, 6th ed. Philadelphia, FA Davis, 1984

2 ▷ Fluid Management and Appropriate Infusates

Key Points

1. General fluid maintenance requirements
2. Goals of fluid therapy and infusates available

General Fluid Maintenance Requirements

Five general points should be considered when providing basic body fluid maintenance requirements:

1. Water
2. Tonicity
3. Other electrolytes
4. pH
5. Calories

Water

The average adult needs between 2000 and 3000 ml of water each day. Normal water losses each day include 600 ml from respiration, 200 ml in feces, 400 ml through perspiration, and approximately 1000 ml to 2000 ml in urine. A general guideline for water replacement is to supply 1500 ml/day/m² of body surface. The patient's body surface measurement in square meters can be easily calculated using a nomogram and the patient's height and weight. If a moderate fluid deficit is present, 2500 ml of water daily per square meter of body surface can be used to correct it; if a severe fluid deficit is present, 3000 ml/day/m² can be administered.

Tonicity

Water is not the only component of body fluid. Certain solute particles must be dissolved in the water to give it the approximate osmolality of actual body fluids. Sodium is the main electrolyte contributing to tonicity, and in general, the amount of sodium needed each day is approximately 100 mEq to 150 mEq. The fluid guideline now becomes: for every square meter of body surface, administer 1500 ml of water and 50 mEq to 75 mEq of sodium daily.

Other Electrolytes

Even though potassium is plentiful within the cells of the body, this stored potassium is not easily accessed. Potassium is usually included in IV fluids at the rate of 50 mEq/1500 ml of water administered. Other electrolytes can usually be disregarded during routine fluid therapy (unless, of course, a specific imbalance is being corrected), since adequate stores of most of the other electrolytes are available and easily accessed by the body.

pH

For routine fluid therapy, the pH of the infusion is not a major consideration. Normal kidneys can easily achieve acid–base balance when given the proper amount of water and the type and amount of electrolytes previously mentioned. Many IV solutions have a pH of about 5.00 because acid solutions have a longer shelf life and are easier to manufacture. Although acid solutions sometimes irritate the walls of veins during administration, normally functioning kidneys can easily buffer the additional acid from the fluid so blood pH won't be affected.

Calories

Most average adults expend approximately 2500 calories each day, more than that if they are stressed or doing heavy exercise, and fewer than that if they are inactive.

Because protein is an important source of calories, a certain amount of daily protein intake is required: approximately 0.5 g to 1g/kg/day is recommended. Most IV maintenance fluids provide only for a state of "semistarvation" by including a few hundred calories in the form of sugar. While that is usually enough to allow for protein sparing in the average patient who will be receiving IV therapy for a short time, patients needing long-term therapy should be evaluated for nutritional status and started on other modalities of nutritional support, such as parenteral nutrition (PN). See Unit IV for a complete discussion.

Goals of Fluid Therapy and Infusates Available

It is the role of the physician to determine both the need for fluid therapy and the appropriate type of fluid therapy. It is the nurse's role to administer the prescribed fluid therapy and also to assess and monitor the patient's fluid status before, during, and after therapy.

Goal 1 of Fluid Therapy

Provide patients with normal maintenance requirements as discussed in the previous section. The general guideline is 1500 ml of water, 50 mEq to 75 mEq of sodium, and 50 mEq of potassium each day per square meter of body surface. This is used as a rough guideline by physicians, since patients must be evaluated on an individual basis. Those with fluid deficit will need more than 1500 ml/day, and those having fluid excess will need far less. Caloric needs can be adjusted accordingly.

Goal 2 of Fluid Therapy

Identify any specific body fluid losses that are occurring and institute replacement with the appropriate infusate. In Chapter 1, Table 1-15 lists specific body fluids and their approximate electrolyte content. Some of the IV fluids currently available are classified as follows: water without salt, water and sodium chloride, premixed potassium chloride, balanced solutions, solutions used for acid–base manipulation, plasma substitutes, ampules available for addition to IV fluids, and solutions of nutritional value. The following display, Available IV Fluids, describes these fluids. By comparing the type of fluid that a patient has lost with the content of possible replacement fluids an appropriate infusate can be selected.

Available IV Fluids

Group 1. Water without Salt

Product	Calories per Liter
Water for injection Ⓐ Ⓣ (not to be used alone)	
Dextrose 2.5% injection Ⓐ Ⓣ*	85
Dextrose 5% in water Ⓐ Ⓜ Ⓣ	170
Dextrose 10% in water Ⓐ Ⓜ Ⓣ	340
Invert sugar (travert) 10% Ⓐ Ⓣ	375
Fructose (levugen, levulose) 10% Ⓐ	375

Ⓐ, Abbott; Ⓜ, McGaw; Ⓣ, Travenol

(Pestana C: *Fluids and Electrolytes in the Surgical Patient,* 3rd ed. Baltimore, Williams & Wilkins, 1985)

Continued

Available IV Fluids (continued)

Group 2. Water and Sodium Chloride

Product	Calories	Na	Cl
Dextrose 5% in 0.11% NaCl Ⓜ	170	19	19
Dextrose 5% in 0.2% NaCl Ⓐ Ⓜ Ⓣ	170	34	34
Dextrose 5% and 0.33% NaCl Ⓐ Ⓜ Ⓣ	170	56	56
Sodium chloride 0.45% Ⓐ Ⓜ Ⓣ		77	77
Dextrose 2½% in ½ normal saline Ⓐ Ⓜ Ⓣ	85	77	77
Dextrose 5% in 0.45% NaCl Ⓐ Ⓜ Ⓣ	170	77	77
Dextrose 10% in 0.45% NaCl Ⓜ	340	77	77
Normal saline (0.9% NaCl) Ⓐ Ⓜ Ⓣ		154	154
Dextrose 5% in 0.9% NaCl Ⓐ Ⓜ Ⓣ	170	154	154
Dextrose 10% in saline Ⓐ Ⓜ Ⓣ	340	154	154
Sodium chloride 3% in water Ⓜ Ⓣ*		513	513
Sodium chloride 5% in water Ⓐ Ⓜ Ⓣ*		855	855

The columns under "Concentration per Liter (mEq)" are Na and Cl.

* Hypertonic solutions. Not for regular IV use.

Continued

Available IV Fluids (continued)

Group 3. Premixed Potassium Chloride

Product	Calories	Concentration per Liter (mEq)		
		Na	Cl	K
Dextrose 5%, 0.075% KCl Ⓐ Ⓣ	170		10	10
Dextrose 5%, 0.2% NaCl, 0.075% KCl Ⓐ Ⓣ	170	34	44	
Dextrose 5%, 0.45% NaCl, 0.075% KCl Ⓐ Ⓣ	170	77	87	
Dextrose 5%, 0.15% KCl Ⓐ Ⓣ, Kadalex Ⓜ	170		20	20
Dextrose 5%, 0.2% NaCL, 0.15% KCl Ⓐ Ⓜ Ⓣ	170	34	54	
Dextrose 5%, 0.33% NaCl, 0.15% KCl Ⓣ	170	56	76	
Dextrose 5%, 0.45% NaCl, 0.15% KCl Ⓐ Ⓜ Ⓣ	170	77	97	
0.9% NaCl with 0.15% KCl Ⓣ		154	174	
Dextrose 5%, 0.2% KCl Ⓐ, Kadalex Ⓜ	170		27	27
Dextrose 5% with 0.224% KCl Ⓐ Ⓣ	170		30	30

Continued

Available IV Fluids (continued)

Group 3. Premixed Potassium Chloride

Product	Calories	Concentration per Liter (mEq)		
		Na	Cl	K
Dextrose 5%, 0.2% NaCl, 0.224% KCl Ⓐ Ⓜ Ⓣ	170	34	64	
Dextrose 5%, 0.33% NaCl, 0.224% KCl Ⓣ	170	56	86	
Dextrose 5%, 0.45% NaCl, 0.224% KCl Ⓐ Ⓜ Ⓣ	170	77	107	
Dextrose 5% with 0.3% KCl Ⓐ Ⓣ, Kadalex Ⓜ	170		40	40
Dextrose 5%, 0.2% NaCl, 0.3% KCl Ⓐ Ⓜ Ⓣ	170	34	74	
Dextrose 5%, 0.33% NaCl, 0.3% KCl Ⓣ	170	56	96	
Dextrose 5%, 0.45% NaCl, 0.3% KCl Ⓐ Ⓜ Ⓣ	170	77	117	
0.9% NaCl with 0.3% KCl Ⓣ		154	194	
For mixture with other solutions, *not* for direct intravenous administration:				
KCl injection USP, 14.9% (2 mEq/ml) Ⓜ Ⓣ		2000	2000	

Continued

Available IV Fluids (continued)

Group 4. Balanced Solutions (listed in order of increasing sodium concentration)

Product

Ionosol MB with dextrose 5% (A)
Isolyte-P with 5% dextrose (M)
5% Dextrose with electrolyte 48 (T)
Invert sugar (travert) 5% in electrolyte No. 4 (polionic 1) (T)
Plasma-Lyte 56 in water (T)
Plasma-Lyte 56 in 5% dextrose (T)
Normosol M in 5% dextrose (A)
Plasma-Lyte M with 5% dextrose (T)
Ionosol T with dextrose 5% (A)
Isolyte M with 5% dextrose (M)
Dextrose 5% with electrolyte 75 (T)
Isolyte R with 5% dextrose (M)
Isolyte H with 5% dextrose (M)
Ionosol B with invert sugar 10% (A)
Ionosol B with dextrose 5% (A)
5% Travert with electrolyte No. 2 (T)
10% Travert with electrolyte No. 2 (T)
Multiple electrolyte No. 2 with 5% invert sugar (M)
Multiple electrolyte No. 2 with 10% invert sugar (M)

P is listed on this table as milliequivalents per liter of HPO_4.
Millimoles of P would be one-half.

Ionosol G with invert sugar 10% (A)
Isolyte G with 5% dextrose (M)
Isolyte G with 10% dextrose (M)
Ionosol G with 10% dextrose (A)

| | Concentration per Liter (mEq) | | | | | | | |
Calories	Na	Cl	K	Ca	Mg	P	Acetate	Lactate
177	25	22	20		3	3		23
		24						
194	30	23	15			3		20
5	40	40	13		3		16	
175								
178	40	40	16	5	3		12	12
176	40	40	35			15		20
		48						
175	41	40	16	5	3		24	
170	42	40	13		3		17	
382	54	49	25		5	13		22
178	57	50	25		5	13		25
		56			6	12		
383								
194	58	51	25		6	13		25
382								

Calories	Na	Cl	K	Ammonium
375	60	147	17	71
170	65	150	17	70
340				

Continued

Group 4. Balanced Solutions (listed in order of increasing sodium concentration)

Product

Dextrose 2.5% in ½ lactated Ringer's
(A) (M)

Dextrose 2.5% in ½ lactated Ringer's (T)

Multiple electrolyte No. 1 with 10% invert
sugar (M)

10% Travert with electrolyte No. 1 (T)

Lactated Ringer's (Hartmann's) (A) (M) (T)

Dextrose 5% in lactated Ringer's (A) (M) (T)

Dextrose 10% in lactated Ringer's (M)

Acetated Ringer's (M)

5% Dextrose with acetated Ringer's (M)

Ionosol D-CM (duodenal) (A)

Ionosol D-CM with dextrose 5% (A)

Ionosol D with invert sugar 10% (A)

Plasma-Lyte 148 in water (T)

Normosol R (A)

Isolyte S (M)

Plasma-Lyte 148 in 5% dextrose (T)

Normosol R in 5% dextrose (A)

Isolyte S in 5% dextrose (M)

Plasma-Lyte 148 (T)

Isolyte E (M)

Isolyte E with 5% dextrose (M)

Plasma-Lyte 148 with 5% dextrose (T)

Plasma-Lyte with 10% travert (T)

Ringer's injection USP (A) (M) (T)

Dextrose 5% in Ringer's (A) (M) (T)

All 3
available
with regular
*p*H or
*p*H 7.4

Calories	Na	Cl	K	Ca	Mg	Gluconate	Acetate	Lactate

Calories	Na	Cl	K	Ca	Mg	Gluconate	Acetate	Lactate
89	65	54	2	1				14
		55		1.5				
395	80	64	36	5	3			60
		63						
9	130	109	4	3				28
179								
349								
	130	110	4	3			27	
177								
16	138	108	12	5	3			50
186								
391	138	100	12					50
18	140	98	5		3	23	27	
185								
20	140	98	10	5	3		48	8
		103						
173		103						
		98						
395								
	147	156	4	5				
170								

Continued

Available IV Fluids (continued)

Group 5. Solutions Used for Acid–Base Manipulation

Product	Concentration per Liter (mEq)		
	Na	Cl	Others
Sodium lactate solution M/G Ⓐ Ⓜ Ⓣ	167		Lactate 167
Sodium bicarbonate 5% Ⓜ Ⓣ Ⓐ	595		Bicarbonate 595
Ammonium chloride 2.14% Ⓜ		400	Ammonium 400
Tham solution Ⓐ			

Plasma Substitutes

Product	per Liter (mEq)		
	Calories	Na	Cl
6% Dextran wv and 0.9% sodium chloride Ⓐ		154	154
6% Dextran wv and 5% dextrose Ⓐ	170		
10% LMD wv and 5% dextrose Ⓐ	170		
10% LMD wv and 0.9% sodium chloride Ⓐ		154	154
Hespan, 6% hetastarch in 0.9% sodium chloride*		154	154

* American Critical Care.

Continued

Group 5. Solutions Used for Acid–Base Manipulation

Ampules Available for Addition to IV Fluids

Sodium chloride, 50, 60, 100, 120 mEq	Calcium gluconate, 4.5 mEq
Sodium lactate, 50, 100, 120 mEq	Calcium gluceptate, 4.5 mEq
Sodium bicarbonate, 2.4, 40, 44.6 mEq	Magnesium sulfate, 8 mEq
Potassium chloride, 10, 20, 30, 40, 60 mEq	Zinc chloride, 1 mg/ml
Potassium phosphate, 30 mEq*	Manganese chloride, 0.1 mg/ml
Potassium acetate, 50, 120, mEq	Cupric chloride, 0.4 mg/ml
Ammonium chloride, 120 mEq	Chromic chloride, 4 mcq/ml
Calcium chloride, 13 mEq	Trace elements (zinc, manganese, copper, chromium)

Dextrose, 7.7 g, 10 g, 11.5 g, 20 g, 30 g, 38 g, 40 g, 50 g, 60 g, 70 g

* The amount of phosphorus will vary with the special product. A commonly used form of potassium phosphate has 15 millimoles of P in 30 mEq.

Continued

Group 6. Solutions of Nutritional Value

Product (Carbohydrates)	Approx. Calories	Osmol. mO
7.7% Dextrose Ⓜ	260	390
10% Dextrose Ⓐ Ⓜ Ⓣ	340	505
10% Dextrose, 0.9% NaCl Ⓐ Ⓜ Ⓣ		813
10% Fructose Ⓐ	375	555
10% Invert sugar Ⓐ		
11.5% Dextrose Ⓜ	390	580
Alcohol 5%, dextrose 5% Ⓐ Ⓜ Ⓣ	450	1114
20% Dextrose Ⓐ Ⓜ Ⓣ	680	1010
Isolyte H-900 cals Ⓜ	900	1890
Normosol M-900 cal Ⓐ	957	
30% Dextrose Ⓐ Ⓜ Ⓣ	1020	1515
38% Dextrose Ⓜ	1290	1920
38.5% Dextrose Ⓐ		
40% Dextrose Ⓐ Ⓜ Ⓣ	1360	2020
50% Dextrose Ⓐ Ⓜ Ⓣ	1700	2526
50% Dextrose with electrolyte pattern B Ⓜ		2615
50% Dextrose with electrolyte and 60 mEq/L acetate Ⓜ		2810
50% Dextrose with electrolyte pattern A Ⓜ		2800
50% Dextrose with electrolytes Ⓐ		2917
60% Dextrose Ⓐ Ⓜ Ⓣ	2040	3030
70% Dextrose Ⓐ Ⓜ Ⓣ	2380	3530

(Note, adjacent to Isolyte H-900 / Normosol M-900 rows: Alcohol 4%, Dextrose 5%, Fructose 15%)

Concentration per Liter (mEq)							
Acetate	Glucon.	Na	Cl	K	Ca	Mg	P (mmol)
		154	154				
16		40	49	13		2	
			40			3	
		32	32		9	16	
60	9.6	80	70	40	9.6	16	
	13	84	115	40	10	16	
36		100	140	80		16	48

Continued

Available IV Fluids (continued)

Group 6. Solutions of Nutritional Value

(Fats)

Liposyn 10% Ⓐ
Intralipid 10% (cutter)
Travamulsion 10% Ⓣ
Liposyn 20% Ⓐ
Intralipid 20% (cutter)
Travamulsion 20% Ⓣ

Group 6. Solutions of Nutritional Value

Product (Proteins)	Approx. Calories
Freamine III 3% with electrolytes Ⓜ	120
Aminosyn 3.5% Ⓐ	140
3.5% Travasol M with electrolyte 45 Ⓣ	
Aminosyn 3.5% M Ⓐ	
Aminosyn 5% Ⓐ	200
Aminosyn RF 5.2% Ⓐ	208
Nephramine 5.4% Ⓜ	216
Travasol 5.5% Ⓣ	220
Travasol 5.5% with electrolytes Ⓣ	
Procalamine (3% aminoach) 3% glycerin) Ⓜ	240
Renamin 6.5% Ⓣ	260
6.9% Freamine HBC Ⓜ	276
Aminosyn 7% Ⓐ	280
Aminosyn 7% with electrolytes Ⓐ	
Hepatamine 8% Ⓜ	320
Freamine IV 8.5% Ⓜ	340

Concentration per Liter (mEq)	
Calories	mO
1100	300
	280
2000	340
	330

Concentration per Liter (mEq)							
Approx. Osm. mO	Acetate	Na	Cl	mEq K	Ca	Mg	P (mmol)
405	44	35	40	24		5	3.5
357	46	7					
450	54	25	25	15		5	7.5
460	58	47	40	13		3	3.5
500	86			5.4			
475	105			5.4			
435	44	5	3				
520	35		22				
850	100	70	70	60		10	30
735	47	35	41	24	3	5	3.5
620	57	10	3				
700	105			5.4			
1013	124	70	96	66		10	30
785	62	10	3				10
810	72	10	3				10

Continued

Available IV Fluids (continued)

Group 6. Solutions of Nutritional Value

Product (Proteins)	Approx. Calories
Travasol 8.5% Ⓣ	
Travasol 8.5% with electrolytes Ⓣ	
Aminosyn 8.5% Ⓐ	
Aminosyn 8.5% with electrolytes Ⓐ	
Aminosyn 10% Ⓐ	400
Travasol 10% Ⓣ	
Freamine III 10% Ⓜ	
Freamine III 10% pH 5.3 Ⓜ	

To facilitate comparisons, all concentrations are noted per liter.
have 500 ml, because they are meant to be mixed with other
rous is expressed in millimoles.

Bibliography

Drescher M: The role of total parenteral nutrition in the management of hospital-acquired malnutrition. NITA 7:133, 1984

Metheny NM, Snively WD: Nurses' Handbook of Fluid Balance, 4th ed. Philadelphia, JB Lippincott, 1983

Approx. Osm. mO	Concentration per Liter (mEq)							
	Acetate	Na	Cl	mEq K	Ca	Mg	P (mmol)
860	52		34				
1160	130	70	70	60		10	30
850	90		35	5.4			
1160	142	70	98	66		10	30
1000	148			5.4			
1000	62		40				
950	88	10	2				10
990	138	10	3				

Please note that many of these solutions come in a 1-liter container, but only solutions. Final concentrations will therefore be halved. Note that phospho-

Pestana C: Fluids and Electrolytes in the Surgical Patient, 3rd ed. Baltimore, Williams & Wilkins, 1985

Plumber A: Principles and Practice of Intravenous Therapy. Boston, Little, Brown, & Co, 1982

Stroot VR, Lee CA, Barrett CA: Fluids and Electrolytes: A Practical Approach, 3rd ed. Philadelphia, FA Davis, 1984

3 ▷ Intravascular Equipment

Key Points

1. Description of gravity flow system
2. Types and characteristics of infusate containers
3. Components and types of administration sets
4. Types and characteristics of infusion devices
5. Types and characteristics of pumps and controllers
6. Description of miscellaneous equipment

Description of Gravity Flow System

Knowledge of the types and characteristics of the components of the gravity flow IV infusion system is essential to ensure safe, effective, and efficient delivery of IV therapy to the patient. The gravity flow IV infusion system is defined as an infusion system that is dependent on fluid flow resulting from gravity pressure of the liquid. The force of gravity "pulls down" on the fluid. This force must create a pressure greater than the patient's venous pressure to allow fluid to enter the venous system. That is, the head pressure must be greater than the venous pressure. The IV infusion system has several components, including the fluid (infusate) container, administration set, infusion device, pump/controller, and possibly other equipment. A description of each component follows.

Types and Characteristics
of Infusate Containers

Three primary types of containers are used: glass, plastic, and hard plastic (semirigid).

Glass Containers

Systems employing glass containers operate on a partial vacuum; air must enter the system to promote an even, controlled flow. Glass infusion systems can be closed or open (Fig. 3-1).

Closed System

A system that allows air to enter the bottle through a filter is ''closed'' if the filter is intact, not wet, and not clogged (Ausman, 1984).

Open System

A system that allows air to enter the bottle through a plastic tube (straw vent) in the bottle is ''open.'' Unfiltered air enters the air space inside the container. To ensure optimal functioning of the straw vent, when the system is primed, the drip chamber should be squeezed and released at the same time that the bottle is inverted. It is essential that the straw extend above the fluid level to prevent bubbling of the air through the infusate. Such bubbling increases the risk of contamination. If any organisms or particles enter the system through the air, they come to rest on the fluid surface. The surface tension of the fluid level should not be broken by shaking the container, since such movement would cause the organisms or particles to become mixed in the infusate. Some sources recommend that the final 50 ml of fluid not be infused, since this quantity would contain any organisms that may have entered through the air vent. However, careful consideration should be given to the impact of this policy on measurement of intake and output, as well as calculation and administration of medications and nutritional supplements.

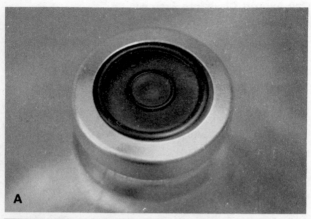

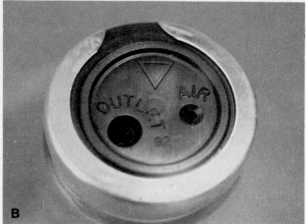

Figure 3-1. *A:* Closed (nonvented) bottle. *B:* Open (vented) bottle.

Types of Glass

Glass containers storing alkaline solutions use *Type I* glass, composed of an expensive substance called borosilicate that minimizes pH changes and glass shedding.

Containers storing acidic or neutral solutions use *Type II* glass, the most common type of glass, composed of dealkalinized glass material and soda lime.

Stoppers

The stopper of glass containers, also called the rubber bung, is composed of numerous substances, including rubber, chemical particles, and cellulose fibers. During insertion of the administration set spike through this bung, coring can occur. That is, visible as well as microscopic particles of the bung can be displaced by the spike and pushed into the IV fluid. This may increase the particulate contamination of the fluid, thereby possibly promoting the development of phlebitis.

Plastic Containers

The majority of IV fluids are packaged in plastic containers (Fig. 3-2). Since the walls of these containers are flexible and collapse as atmospheric pressure pushes on the container to force fluid out, air does not enter the system—it is truly a closed infusion system. A membrane seals both the medication and the administration ports of the container, thus ensuring no entry of air into the system. Most plastic containers are composed of polyvinylchloride (PVC), chemicals that give plastic its flexibility. Numerous studies have looked at the relationship between leaching and PVC. Leaching, the dissolving of plasticizers into the infusate, is possibly associated with increased rates of phlebitis. Since these containers are not impervious to moisture, there is a chance of contamination of the infusate if the container is placed on a wet

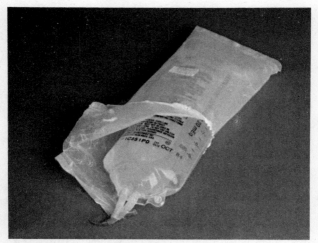

Figure 3-2. Plastic infusion bag.

surface. However, the benefits of using plastic containers appear to far outweigh the risks associated with leaching.

Hard Plastic (Semirigid) Containers

The most recent type of infusate containers to be developed is the semirigid, hard plastic unit (Fig. 3-3). Like the plastic container, the hard plastic container is a truly closed system. It offers the advantage of containing no plasticizers, and the container has marks that make it easy to read fluid levels.

All infusate containers are subject to variable total volumes. The United States Pharmacopeia recommends that infusate containers of 50 ml or more be filled with a 2% to 3% excess (Turco, 1981). This excess volume allows for wetting of container walls, priming of the administration set, and so forth.

The advantages and disadvantages of the major types of infusate containers are summarized in Table 3-1.

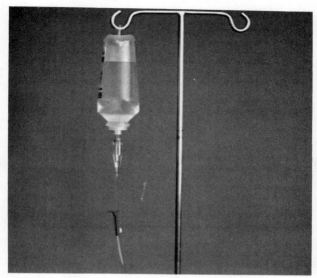

Figure 3-3. Rigid or hard plastic container.

Table 3-1. Advantages and Disadvantages of Glass, Plastic, and Hard Plastic Infusate Containers

	Advantages	**Disadvantages**
Glass	Rigid construction promotes ease of handling	Possible hairline cracks and other imperfections in container difficult to see
	Withstands internal pressure	Heavy weight
	Inert; has no plasticizers	Cumbersome disposal
	Fluid level easily read	Requires air to enter system, possibly increasing contamination
	Clear container facilitates inspection	Rubber bung increases particulate contamination

Table 3-1.   (Continued)

	Advantages	Disadvantages
Glass (cont.)		Complete container includes both glass and rubber and, possibly, plastic components, increasing compatibility concerns
		Easily broken if displaced from IV pole
Plastic	Closed system	Punctures easily
	Flexible	Fluid level determination difficult
	Lightweight	
	Unbreakable	Chances of contamination if placed on wet surface due to permeability of plastic
	Ideal for infusion under pressure	
	Complete container composed of one substance, minimizing incompatibility concerns	Composed of plasticizers that may increase particulate matter
		Not completely inert; leaching of plasticizers and adsorption of substances to surface can occur
		Used in a series with other similar containers, may promote movement of residual air into IV line
Hard Plastic (semirigid)	Closed system	Used in a series with other similar containers, may promote movement of residual air into IV line
	Fluid level easy to determine	
	Lightweight	
	Unbreakable	
	Plastic material inert	
	Impermeable to moisture	

Components and Types of Administration Sets

The administration set is used to deliver the infusate from the IV container to the patient. Several types are used. Following a review of the components of a standard set, the major categories of administration sets are briefly described.

Components of the Administration Set

See Figure 3-4 for illustration of each component.

Spike/Piercing Pin. The spike/piercing pin (Fig. 3-5) is a sharply tipped plastic tube designed to be inserted into the infusate container. It connects to the drop orifice.

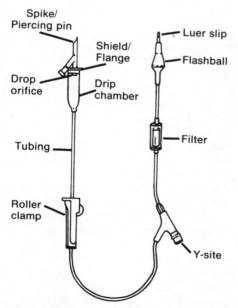

Figure 3-4. Components of the administration set.

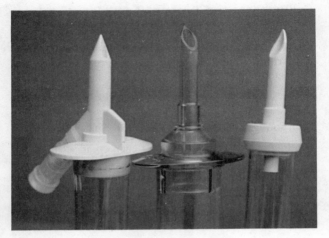

Figure 3-5. Infusion container spikes.

Shield/Flange. The shield/flange is a plastic guard that helps prevent touch contamination during insertion of the spike (spiking).

Drop Orifice. Found near the proximal end of the administration set, the drop orifice is an opening that determines the size and shape of the fluid drop that can be produced by the administration set.

Drip Chamber. The drip chamber is a pliable, enlarged plastic tube that contains the drop orifice. It is connected to the tubing at its outlet.

Tubing. A length of plastic tubing connects the drip chamber to a connector and consequently an infusion device. Depending on the manufacturer, the tubing may have a variety of clamps, ports, connectors, and filters included.

Clamp. The clamp is a flow control device that operates on the principle of compression of the tubing wall to change the diameter of the tube, thereby altering flow rate. Three common types of clamps are roller, screw, and slide (Fig. 3-6). All operate on the same principle of

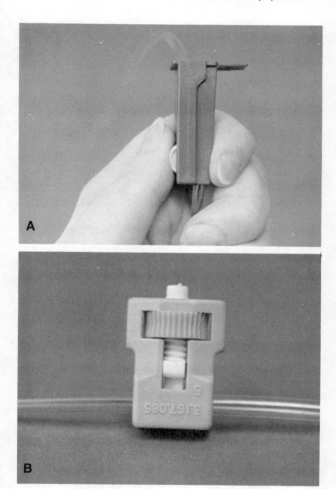

Figure 3-6. *A:* Roller clamp. *B:* Screw clamp. *C:* Slide clamp.

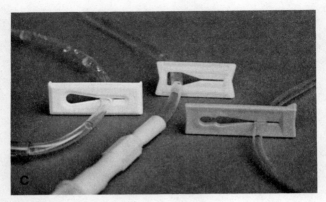

Figure 3-6. (Continued)

compression. The roller and screw clamps are viewed as equally reliable. The slide clamp may be less reliable in controlling flow.

Injection Ports. The injection ports serve as access sites into the tubing and can be located at various points along the administration set. Examples can include Y-type and T-type devices, stopcocks, and flashballs. They are used for medication administration. Special attention should be given to the dead space volumes of these sites. These can alter the actual amount of solution administered (Arwood et al, 1982). Small needles (21–25 gauge) should be used for injecting into these ports to ensure resealing.

Final Filter. The final filter removes foreign particles from the infusion fluid. (Fig. 3-7). It can be purchased as an integral part of the administration set tubing or can be used as an add-on feature when assembling a set. Filter functions may include the following:

- Particulate matter removal
- Air elimination
- Endotoxin retention
- Pressure protection

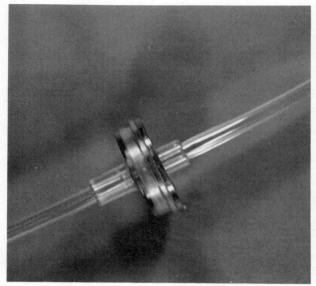

Figure 3-7. Filter.

Depending on composition materials, filters can adsorb (bind) drugs to their membrane, thus reducing the amount of medication available to the patient. Two filter pore sizes are available: the 0.45-μm filter traps particulates, fungi, and most bacteria; the 0.22-μm filter traps particulates, fungi, and all bacteria. Filters are of two basic structures: membrane filters and depth filters.

1. Membrane filters, which trap particles on the surface of the filter, can clog easily and impede flow if used to filter a solution heavy with particulate matter.
2. Depth filters trap particles within the filter material itself. Fluid flow is usually easier to maintain through these filters because there is more available material in which to trap particles without occluding the entire membrane.

Use of final filter includes the following advantages:

- They remove almost all particulate matter.
- They usually prevent air embolism.
- They can decrease phlebitis incidence.
- They are cost-effective (Rutherford, 1985).

Use of final filters include the following disadvantages:

- They are air locking.
- They are filter clogging.
- They are drug binding.

It has been recommended that final filters be used for the following:

- Patients who are immunocompromised
- Patients who are receiving total parenteral nutrition (TPN)
- Patients receiving solutions that contain many additives such as cephalosporins, penicillin G potassium, and ampicillin sodium
- Neonates

Flashball. A rubber bulb (Fig. 3-8), located between the end of the tubing and the connector end, is used to observe backflow of blood during insertion of the infusion device (described in Chapter 7) and as a delivery port for IV medication and fluid by syringe puncture, as described in Chapter 14.

Connector/Lock. The connector/lock device is attached to the end of the tubing, allowing a tight connection between tubing and the infusion device. Examples are Luer slip lock, Click Lock, and Piggy Mate IV Tubing Lock (Intravenous Therapy News, 1985). Selection criteria for connectors and locks should ensure that they (Kleeman, 1985):

- Are safe, simple, and inexpensive
- Fit smoothly against the skin
- Offer universality of fit

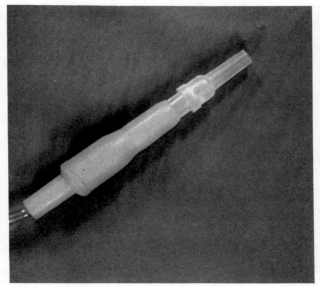

Figure 3-8. Flashball.

- Do not interfere with the angle of the catheter
- Are able to be disconnected easily and quickly

Types of Administration Sets

Continuous Administration Sets

1. *Standard administration set.* The standard (regular) administration set (Fig. 3-9) is calibrated to deliver between 10 and 20 gtt (drops)/ml depending on the individual manufacturer (Table 3-2). The calibration for each specific set can be found in the accompanying manufacturer's literature. These sets are routinely used for infusion when additional equipment is not needed for medication administration. During admin-

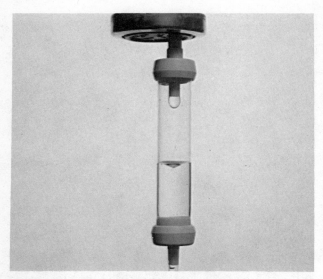

Figure 3-9. Standard (regular) administration set.

istration of medications, the solution may layer in this larger-intraluminal-diameter tubing, thus prolonging the drug delivery time and the onset and completion of drug infusions (Leff and Roberts, 1985).

2. *Minidrop and microdrop.* This administration set is calibrated to deliver 60 gtt/ml. This is accomplished by reducing the size of the drop. These sets are used when relatively small amounts of fluid are to be ad-

Table 3-2. Calibration of Standard Infusion Sets

Type of Set	Abbott	Cutter	McGaw	Travenol
Standard (gtt/ml)	15	20	15	10
Minidrop (gtt/ml)	60	60	60	60

ministered over a relatively long time or to run an infusion at a keep-open rate.

3. *Low-volume IV tubing*. This administration tubing, possessing a small intraluminal diameter of 0.06 cm to 0.14 cm, is used for medication administration. Use of this tubing greatly reduces the time required for onset and completion of drug infusion and minimizes layering of medication within the tubing.

Intermittent Administration Sets

Intermittent sets are used primarily for the administration of medications. Types of sets include the following:

1. *Secondary/add-a-line*. Secondary or add-a-line sets include a primary line with a check valve and a secondary set composed of any size infusate container. Both infusate containers hang at the same level; the secondary set connects to the primary set at some lower Y port (secondary port) on the primary line. A valve on the primary line ensures infusion of only the primary infusate or the secondary solution at one time and allows the primary solution flow to resume automatically following infusion of the secondary infusion.

2. *Piggyback lines*. Piggyback lines may or may not include a check valve as part of the primary line. The secondary set consists of a 50-ml to 100-ml infusate container and short tubing (usually standard drip). The primary infusate is positioned lower than the secondary container, using an extension hook provided. The secondary tubing connects to the primary line at an upper Y port piggyback port.

3. *Volume-controlled sets*. This specifically designed set allows for intermittent administration of measured volumes of fluid with a calibrated chamber or burette. These sets are also used for volume control in both children and adults. One example is a set that consists of a series of small plastic chambers. Another type is the calibrated burette chamber (Fig. 3-10).

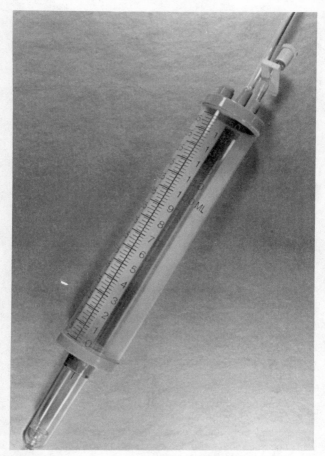

Figure 3-10. Calibrated burette chamber.

Types and Characteristics of Infusion Devices

Several types of infusion devices are used, depending on whether peripheral or central venous infusion sites are chosen. A summary of the advantages and disadvantages of each site is included in Table 3-3.

Table 3-3. Advantages and Disadvantages of
Peripheral or Central Sites

	Advantages	Disadvantages
Peripheral	Used for administration of isotonic fluids	Become irritated with administration of hypertonic fluids
	Appropriate for short-term therapy	Require frequent change of site
	Can be used for alert, oriented patients	Can be removed by disoriented patients
	Used for administration of nonirritating medications	Cannot provide appropriate dilution of irritating medications
Central	Can be used for administration of hypertonic infusate	Possibly promote a greater number of systemic complications
	Appropriate for long-term therapy	
	Less accessible to the disoriented patient's attempts at removal	Insertion requires absolute cooperation of patient
	Used for administration of irritating substances	Possibly associated with greater risk of complications such as shock

Selection of the appropriate infusion device is influenced by the following:

- Patient age
- Condition of vessels
- Diagnosis
- Length of therapy
- Frequency of administration
- Volume of infusate
- Type of infusate or medication

Peripheral Infusion Devices

Steel Needles
Examples of steel needles include scalp-vein or winged-tip needles (Fig. 3-11). Metal needles are ½ to 2 inches in

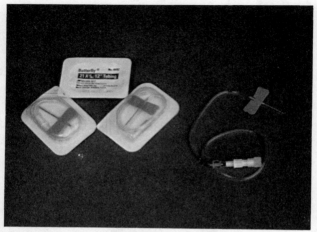

Figure 3-11. Winged-tip steel needle.

length and range from 14 to 25 gauge; some are attached to 3 to 12 inches of plastic tubing. They are commonly used for infants, children, and the elderly for short-term (single-dose or less than 24-hour) therapy, to administer IV push medication, or to obtain blood samples. Winged units provide greater stability. They cannot be used with some forms of chemotherapy, since the medication interacts with the aluminum alloy. Some metal needles are coated with silicone, which is believed to reduce thrombus formation (Coco, 1980). The use of steel needles may result in lower infective complications, but may also limit the patient's mobility by being rigid. They may cause more discomfort than other infusion devices.

Over-the-Needle Plastic Infusion Device

The over-the-needle radiopaque plastic infusion device, commonly called a cannula or catheter, ranges from 1/4 to 5 1/2 inches in length and from 14 to 24 gauge. It can be composed of various plastic materials, including silicone, Teflon, PVC, or polyethylene, and is fused to a rigid hub. The needle is used for venipuncture, then removed (Fig.

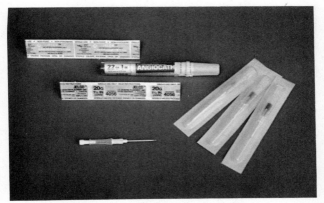

Figure 3-12. Over-the-needle catheter.

3-12). It is used for the unstable, restless, or agitated patient, one with poor sites, for the administration of irritating or large-volume solutions, and in both long-term and short-term therapy. Since it is pliable, it is comfortable and less likely to puncture the vessel wall on movement. Using a sterile adapter plug, the cannula can be converted to a heparin lock.

Through-the-Needle Plastic Infusion Device
A plastic catheter, 8 to 36 inches in length, is inserted through a separate needle (Fig. 3-13). In certain types of catheters, once introduced, the needle remains over a segment of the catheter; in other types, complete removal of the needle is possible after the catheter is inserted. It is used for administration into a central vein, when peripheral veins are difficult to access, for long-term therapy, and for infusion of very irritating solutions.

Heparin Locks
Although usually a steel needle with a rubber injection cap, the heparin lock can also consist of an adapter having a rubber injection cap applied to the plastic cannula

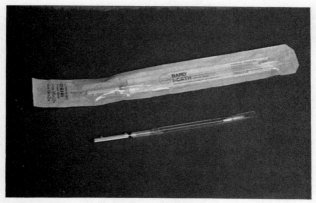

Figure 3-13. Through-the-needle catheter.

(Fig. 3-14). It is used for short-term and intermittent delivery of fluids and medications in stable patients. Patency is maintained by instilling weak heparin or saline solution. Complications per patient-day have been shown to be lower than with continuous infusions (Hanson, 1976).

Central Venous Infusion Devices

(See Chapter 11 for further details.)

Central Catheter

Usually ranging from 15 to 18 gauge and from 15 cm to 30 cm in length, the central catheter is a silicone elastomer or polyurethane device inserted into the subclavian or jugular vein and advanced into the large superior vena cava.

Peripherally Inserted Central Venous Catheter

Usually averaging 15 gauge and 50 cm to 60 cm in length, the peripheral catheter is inserted into a peripheral site

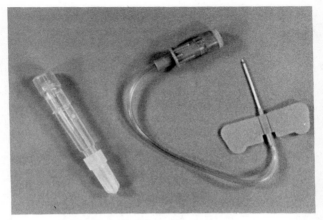

Figure 3-14. Heparin lock infusion devices.

(*e.g.*, cephalic or basilic vein) and advanced into the superior vena cava.

Hickman Catheter
The Hickman catheter is a 90-cm-long, 1.6-mm-diameter, silicone Silastic, long-term dwelling catheter equipped with one or two Dacron cuffs. It allows for central drawing of blood samples (Fig. 3-15).

Broviac Catheter
The Broviac device is a 90-cm-long, 1.0-mm-diameter silicone Silastic long-term dwelling catheter equipped with cuffs. It allows for infusion of IV fluids including parenteral nutrition.

Double-Lumen Hickman (Hickman–Broviac) Catheter
A Hickman and a Broviac catheter, fused together, is placed into a large vein with the tip resting in the right atrium. It allows for long-term venous access for the purposes of fluid replacement, nutrition, blood and medication administration, and blood drawing.

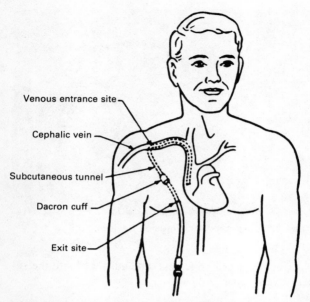

Figure 3-15. Hickman catheter (Metheny N: Fluid and Electrolyte Balance, p 129. Philadelphia, JB Lippincott, 1987).

Groshong Catheter

The Groshong catheter is a thin-walled silicone rubber catheter constructed with a two-way slit valve located at the tip. Although it is similar to the Hickman catheter, its design allows for both fluid administration and blood sampling through the same lumen.

Implantable Venous Access Ports

A completely closed system composed of an implanted device consisting of a drug reservoir, or port, with a self-sealing system connected to an outlet catheter is surgically implanted in a subcutaneous pocket at a convenient body site. Used for long-term therapy, this device decreases the possibility of drug infiltration, vein sclerosis, and infection.

Types and Characteristics of Pumps and Controllers

Electronic infusion devices can be used to control the flow rate of an infusion. Use of electronic infusion devices provide the advantages of maintaining more accurate flow rates, decreasing the number of IV flow checks by nurses, decreasing IV therapy–related morbidity, and allowing for intra-arterial administration of drugs. Disadvantages of these devices include that they may be complicated to use, may require time to prepare, may require special training of personnel, may be costly to purchase, and may create a false sense of security for nursing staff.

Controllers

Controllers regulate the flow (head pressure) created by gravity (Fig. 3-16). They control flow but do not exert pressure. Controllers are governed by the same flow

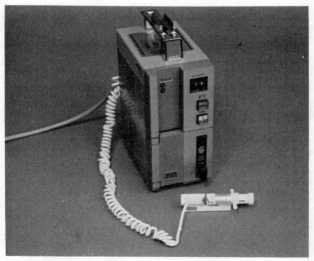

Figure 3-16. Controller.

properties as the gravity flow system. Controllers can be volumetric or nonvolumetric.

1. *Volumetric controllers.* Calibrated to infuse a specific volume at a specific rate, volumetric controllers are more accurate than nonvolumetric controllers. Examples include IVAC 260 and 600, IMED 922 and 927, Quest Med, DNA Flo Control, Centaur Guardian II, Simplicity 2100A, Valley Lab 5000 B, and Anattos Dateminder.
2. *Nonvolumetric controllers.* Nonvolumetric controllers are calibrated to infuse at a specified drop rate. Infusion is based on drops per minute, not volume per minute. Examples include IVAC 230, Travenol 3000, Flo-Gard, McGaw Epic Controller, IMED 350, and DELMED Tru-Flo.

Pumps

Electronic infusion devices that exert positive pressure to influence flow rate are pumps (Fig. 3-17). This positive pressure is measured in pounds per square inch (psi) of millimeters of mercury. The pressure exerted must be appropriate for the in-line filter being used and enough to

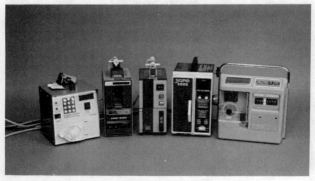

Figure 3-17. Infusion pump.

overcome the venous or arterial pressure, depending on the infusion site.

1. *Volumetric pumps.* Calibrated to infuse a specific volume at a specific rate, volumetric pumps include rotary, linear, roller peristaltic, piston-syringe (cassette), and syringe types. Figure 3-18 illustrates a syringe pump. These are more accurate than nonvolumetric pumps. Examples include IMED 928, 929, 960, and 965; IVAC 560, 630, and 1500; Travenol Flo-Gard 6000 and 8000; Life Care Model 3; Cutter Dependo Flo; Critikon 2100A; Sigma 5000; Valley Lab 6000 and 6006; and AVI Guardian 1000.
2. *Nonvolumetric pumps.* Calibrated to infuse at a specified drop rate, nonvolumetric pumps include the IVAC 530 peristaltic.

Description of Miscellaneous Equipment

Pressure Infusion Sleeve

The pressure infusion sleeve is a commercially available sleeve with a pneumatic cuff into which the plastic infusate container is placed. The pressure that is created by

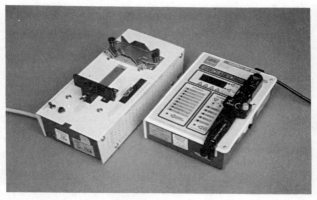

Figure 3-18. Syringe pump.

inflating the cuff promotes more rapid infusion of the fluid or infusion of the fluid against arterial pressure.

Fluid Warmer
The fluid warmer is a device used for warming parenteral fluids, including blood. It serves as a means of minimizing body heat loss or the effects of hypothermia (Gough, 1985).

Tourniquets
Tourniquets include rubber tubing, a Velcro strap, or use of the blood pressure cuff.

Site-Cleansing Supplies
Iodine, iodophore, povidone-iodine, chlorhexidine, and 70% alcohol wipes or swabs are used to clean the site.

Tapes
Tape includes paper, nonallergic, or adhesive varieties.

Stabilization/Anchoring Devices
Anchoring devices are used to secure and minimize movement of the infusion device or limb.

Dressings
Categories include sterile gauze and transparent/occlusive dressings.

Antiseptic Ointments
Antiseptics are occasionally used at insertion sites to inhibit growth of microorganisms. Examples are polyantimicrobic or iodine base.

Flow Control Devices
Flow control attachments to the gravity flow administration set may assist in monitoring the drop rate/flow. Examples include Accudrop (Accudrop, 1984) and STASET (Beckton-Dickinson, Rutherford, NJ).

Plastic Loop

A preformed section of tubing, one end of which is attached to the infusion device and the other end to the administration tubing, may help secure tubing and prevent kinks.

Specialized Equipment

(See Chapter 13 for further discussion of equipment related to hemodynamic monitoring, Chapter 14 for further discussion of equipment related to administration of medications, Chapter 15 for further discussion of equipment related to administration of blood, and Chapter 16 for further discussion of specialized equipment used in home IV therapy.)

Bibliography

Accudrop™. NITA 7(3):244, 1984

Armstrong E, Bailie M: Clinical comparison of three volumetric infusion pumps. NITA 8(4):305, 1985

Arwood L, Anderson C, Cardero L et al: The effect of intravenous tubing internal radius and injection port position in drug delivery. Clin Res 30:790A, 1982

Ausman RK: Intravascular Infusion Systems, pp 16 and 17. Hingham, MA, MTP Press, 1984

Chrystal C: Volumetric pump or controller? NITA Update, 5:3, 1984

Coco C: Intravenous Therapy. St Louis, CV Mosby, 1980

Coggin S: Evaluating and selecting I.V. equipment. NITA 10(1):52, 1987

Gill S: Is filtration cost-effective in routine IV therapy? NITA 7:227, 1984

Gough J: I.V. fluid warmers show clinical utility for hypothermia outside OR. Parenterals 3(1):103, 1985

Hanson R: Heparin-lock or keep open IV? Am J Nur 76:1102, 1976

Harrigan C: Care and cost justification of final filtration. NITA 8:426, 1985

Intravenous therapy news. Pharmacy Practice News 12(11): 3, 1985

Kleeman A: Our patients deserve better IV locks. RN, 48:16–17, 1985

Leff R, Roberts R: Practical Aspects of Intravenous Drug Therapy Techniques. Bethesda, MD, American Society of Hospital Pharmacists, 1985

Metheny N: Fluid and Electrolyte Balance, p 129. Philadelphia, J B Lippincott, 1987

Newton R, DeYoung J, Levin H: Volumes of implantable vascular access devices and heparin flush requirements. NITA 8(1):137, 1985

Rutherford C: Cost-effectiveness of filters. NITA Update 6(2):5, 1985

Turco S: Excess fills in parenterals. Am J Intravenous Ther Clin Nutr 8(1):7, 1981

Turco S: Mechanical and electronic equipment for parenteral and enteral use: and update. NITA Update 2(4):1, 1984

4 ▷   Flow Factors in Intravenous Therapy

Key Points

1. Principles of flow in the gravity flow system
2. Components of the IV administration system that influence flow
3. Components of the venous system that influence flow

Principles of Flow in the Gravity Flow System

Flow in the gravity infusion system is dependent on the interplay between a pressure gradient and the opposing resistance. A pressure gradient consists of an area of higher pressure and an area of lower pressure. In the IV system the pressure of the infusate must be greater than the pressure in the venous system in order for the IV fluid to move into the venous system. Resistance is any factor that slows or impedes this flow. The total amount of resistance must be less than total pressure for infusate flow to occur. Each component of the IV administration system can influence the flow.

Components of the IV Administration System That Influence Flow

Infusate Container

Head pressure decreases as the container empties, thus decreasing flow. Air vent (straw tube) obstruction may decrease flow.

Infusate

Increases in viscosity or density of the fluid decrease flow. The temperature of the solution and of the room may alter flow. The greater the height of the infusate, the greater the gravity pressure promoting flow. Height of the infusate, which influences flow, is affected by the fluid level in the container, the height of the bed, and the position of the IV pole. Additives may alter the flow of the infusate by changing its specific gravity and surface tension. Cohesion, the attraction between molecules of a substance, may also alter flow rate; the greater the cohesion, the slower the flow, and vice versa.

Drop Orifice (Drop Chamber)

The size of the drop orifice, standard drop vs. minidrop, determines the amount of fluid volume in each drop. Since defects and irregularities in the orifice can change moistening of that orifice, the actual volume of the drops may be altered up to 40%. Metal drop orifices found in the minidrop administration sets have fewer irregularities in drop formation (La Cour, 1965).

The rate of drop formation at the orifice also influences flow. The drop size for both macrodrop and microdrop sets may increase as much as 25% during rapid administration. That is, drops flowing at a fast rate are bigger (hold more infusate) than drops flowing at a slow rate (Ferenchak et al, 1971). It is important to note that administration rates based on drops per minute are at best an estimate of the quantity of fluid delivered.

Shunting, which is the flow of fluid down the chamber wall rather than the dropping of fluid from the drop orifice into the chamber, leads to erratic flow that is difficult to regulate. If this occurs, it is best to replace the set.

Tubing

The greater the diameter of the tubing, the less resistance, therefore the greater the flow. Air, kinks, constrictions, irregularities, and pinched or disconnected areas in the tubing decrease fluid flow.

Clamp

Creeping, or cold flow, a change in the inside diameter of the tubing that occurs within half an hour after the clamp has been set, changes the flow rate. In addition, wear and tear on the tubing caused by the pressure of the clamp can alter the flow of the fluid. Slippage, or unintentional opening of the clamp, is another concern in regulating flow of infusate through the tubing. Several administration sets have shown more than a 15% change in rate within 45 minutes the initial setting owing to slippage (Ziser et al, 1979). Slippage occurs every time the clamp is moved to a different area on the tubing.

Metal Needle/Cannula/Catheter

The greater the gauge number of the infusion device, the smaller its diameter and, consequently, the less flow possible. If the bevel rests against the vessel wall, flow is decreased. Following placement in the venous system, flow through the plastic cannula or catheter may be decreased somewhat because of the development of fibrin sleeves. These sleeves may form on interior and exterior surfaces of the infusion device within 20 to 30 minutes. This can be due to the wetability characteristics, the electrical charge, and surface irregularities of the device. In addition, damaged platelets or platelet contact with collagen exposed during catheter insertion can initiate the formation of these sleeves (Jacobsson and Schlossman, 1969; Nachnani et al, 1972; Nejad et al, 1968).

Filters and Ancillary Devices

The addition of any component to the administration system will increase resistance and thus decrease flow. Filters can become air locked, thus occluding flow. Tape that is applied too tightly can pinch tubing and restrict flow.

Components of the Venous System
That Influence Flow

Patient's Blood Pressure

The level of venous pressure determines the amount of gravity pressure required to create flow into the venous system. The higher the venous blood pressure, the greater the gravity pressure must be to cause fluid to enter the vein and vice versa. Blood pressure, then, always influences flow rate.

Venous Spasm

Pain, irritation, a change in temperature of the infusate, or the patient's emotional response to fear can cause a vasovagal response leading to venous spasms. As the vein constricts or relaxes, the venous resistance to infusate flow alters the flow rate.

Blood Viscosity

The greater the blood viscosity (the higher the hematocrit), the greater its resistance to the flow of infusate.

Size of the Vessel

Larger veins, by offering less resistance, permit greater flow. Likewise, smaller veins create more resistance against the flow of infusing fluid.

Vein/Infusion Device Ratio

If the needle, cannula, or catheter is so large as to almost fill the vein, flow of the patient's blood through the vein can be impeded, therefore slowing the flow of infusate into the vein. If a very small needle, cannula, or catheter is placed in a much larger vessel, the patient's blood flow through the veins can slow or prevent the flow of infusate from entering the vein from the administration set.

Placement of Needle/Cannula/Catheter

The mere placement of the infusion device into the vein disrupts the smooth, laminar flow pattern that is characteristic of normal blood flow. This interruption causes the flow to become turbulent. A combination of the turbulent blood flow and the infusion device placement causes blood platelets to move from their usual position near red blood cells flowing in the center of the blood vessel to a new position next to the vessel wall. This movement may cause damage to the platelets, which can result in some clotting (thrombus formation) that will impede infusate flow to the vein. It is important, then, that the infusion device be adequately stabilized.

Multiple factors influencing flow rate have been discussed. In addition, the patient's activity level and overall condition can have an impact on flow.

Bibliography

Boothe C, Talley J: Mechanical and electronic intravenous infusion devices, part I. Infusion 10(1):6, 1986

Ferenchak P, Collins J, Morgan A: Drop size and rate in parenteral infusion. Surgery 70:674, 1971

Gurevich I: Are I.V. in-line filters worth the price? Nursing 86 16:42–43, 1986

Jacobsson B, Schlossman D: Angiographic investigation of formation of thrombi on vascular catheters. Radiology 93:355, 1969

LaCour D: Drop size in disposable sets for intravenous infusion. Acta Anaesthesiol Scand 9:145, 1965

Nachnani G, Lessin L, Motomiya T et al: Scanning electron microscopy of thrombogenesis on vascular catheter surfaces. N Engl J Med 286:139, 1972

Nejad M, Klaper M, Steggerda F et al: Clotting on the outer surfaces of vascular catheters. Radiology 91:248, 1968

Store R: Current concepts of flow control. NITA 7(6):517, 1984

Talley J: Mechanical and electronic intravenous infusion devices, part II. Infusion 10(2):31, 1986

Ziser M, Freezor M, Skolaut M: Regulating intravenous fluid flow: Controller vs clamps. Am J Hosp Pharm 36:1090, 1979

Unit II

Nursing Interventions: Techniques and Procedures of Intravenous Therapy

5 ▷ Initiating Intravenous Therapy

Key Points

1. Physician's order
2. Patient assessment
3. Handwashing
4. Patient identification
5. Psychological preparedness
6. Infusion selection and preparation
7. Vein selection
8. Needle/cannula selection
9. Vein dilatation methods
10. Preinsertion local anesthesia
11. Site preparation
12. Vein entry
13. Stabilization
14. Topical ointments
15. Dressings
16. Flow rate
17. Charting

Physician's Order

1. Evaluate the IV order for the following:
   - Solution name
   - Solution volume
   - Rate of administration
   - Directions for subsequent administration of fluids
2. If the infusate is to include a medication, the following should be noted in the order:
   - Unabbreviated name of the medication
   - Exact dosage

- Exact route of administration
- Frequency of administration

Patient Assessment

Document current status of the patient by completing or reviewing the nursing history and physical assessment. Particularly note any allergies to infusates, medications, iodine, or tape. Review reason and goal/outcome for IV therapy.

Handwashing

1. Hospital personnel should wash their hands for at least 15 to 20 seconds before equipment preparation (Fig. 5-1), before insertion, following the procedure, and prior to and following any contact with the patient or the equipment.
2. Soap and water is adequate for most peripheral insertions, but an antiseptic soap containing chemicals such as iodine or chlorhexidine should be used before

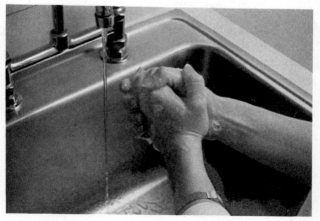

Figure 5-1. Wash hands for 15-20 seconds prior to preparing equipment.

insertion of central cannulas or cannulas requiring a cutdown.

3. Do not use hand lotion following handwashing.
4. Avoid wearing false fingernails, which can increase the number of hand-carried microorganisms (Infection traced to false fingernails, 1985).

Patient Identification

Properly identify the patient.

Psychological Preparedness

1. Evaluate the psychological preparedness of the patient. Psychologically, IV therapy may mean the following:
   - Decreased independence
   - Decreased autonomy
   - Invasion of personal space
   - Increased fear and anxiety related to pain, air infusion, germs and infection, concern about mistakes in delivery and equipment failure, and lack of understanding related to the necessity for the therapy
2. Minimize fear and anxiety by instructing the patient as to the following:
   - What an IV is
   - Reason for the IV
   - The procedure
   - What is infused
   - What to do to maintain the IV
3. Provide privacy.
4. Provide comfort.
5. Assess possible implications of religious beliefs for IV therapy. Examples include the following:
   - Jehovah's Witnesses do not believe in blood transfusion or administration of blood products; this does not apply to artificial red blood cells.
   - Christian Scientists may refuse any form of medical assistance.

• Some persons believe that admission of pain is a
weakness and may indicate lack of faith; that pain
and suffering are God's punishment for their sins;
that by enduring pain they can transcend their
bodies and attain a higher state of being.

Infusion Selection and Preparation

Infusate Container

1. Inspect for discoloration, cloudiness, foreign matter.
2. Inspect glass containers for cracks by rotating in
   light.
3. Inspect plastic bags for pinholes by gently squeezing
   the container.
4. Inspect seals to ensure they are intact.
5. Listen for indications of the presence of a vacuum
   when removing the seal of glass containers.
6. Review expiration date.
7. Check for correct type of solution.
8. Label correctly by including date, time, initials of the
   person initiating the flow, and flow schedule, if applicable.
9. Complete equipment preparation in a quiet area with
   least amount of traffic and air currents. Increased
   traffic and air currents could contribute to increased
   contamination rates.
10. Ensure that all surfaces coming in contact with the
    plastic infusate container are dry.
11. Avoid vigorous shaking of the plastic infusate con-
    tainer since this can increase levels of particulate
    matter (Darby and Ausman, 1974).

Selection of Infusion Set

The infusion system selected should do the following
(Chrystal, 1985):

1. Deliver the prescribed therapy while minimizing the
   risk of infection
2. Minimize the number of connection points in the
   setup

3. Minimize cost to the patient
4. Ensure that incompatible drugs are never administered through the same tubing
5. Include appropriate final filtration devices

Spiking and Priming a Basic Infusion Set

Spiking is defined as inserting the administration set into the infusate container. *Priming* is defined as filling the administration set with infusate for the first time.

The procedure for spiking and priming of the basic infusion set includes the following steps:

1. Wash hands, assemble equipment, and maintain sterility throughout the procedure.
2. Locate the clamp just below the drip chamber.
3. Close the clamp.
4. Remove the protective cover over the piercing pin.
5. Remove the protective seal from the IV container. (If the infusate container is a vented bottle, remove the latex cover and listen for the hissing sound that ensures the vacuum seal of the bottle.)
6. Push the spike firmly into the stopper or port while ensuring that no touch contamination of the spike or port occurs. If spiking the plastic bag, hang the bag before inserting the spike using a twisting motion. If spiking a vented bottle, insert the spike into the larger of the two holes.
7. Fill the drop chamber to one-half full by squeezing the walls.
8. Flush the tubing by releasing the clamp while holding the unfilled tubing higher than the filled portion. By allowing the fluid to "run up" the tubing, air bubbles are not trapped near the tubing walls but are forced to move throughout the length of the tubing and be expelled. Depending on the manufacturer, flushing may require between 5 and 15 ml.
9. Hang the primed infusion set 36 to 45 inches above the infusion site.
10. Label the tubing indicating the date, time, and initials

of the person adding the set. Place label immediately
distal to the clamp device.

Spiking and Priming a Piggyback Infusion Set

Spike and prime the secondary infusion, piggyback, set
by performing the following steps:

1. Swab the Y site of the primary set with alcohol.
2. Insert the needle of the secondary set into the Y site.
3. Backprime the secondary set by lowering the secondary solution container until the drip chamber of the secondary set is one-half full.
4. Establish the flow by opening the clamp of the secondary bag.
5. Label the tubing indicating the date, time, and initials of the person adding the set.

Vein Selection

1. Evaluate the clinical condition of the patient by the following assessment:
    • Is the patient stable/unstable?
    • Is there a likelihood of the patient experiencing shock?
    • Is the patient alert or confused?
    • What is the purpose of the infusion?
    • Will medications be administered intravenously?
    • What type of solution will be administered?
    • Is short-term or long-term therapy required?
    • What clinical procedures are anticipated?
    • What site does the patient state is best?
2. Evaluate the comfort of the patient by the following assessment:
    • What site does the patient prefer?
    • What arm/hand is dominant?
    • What degree of mobility is desired?
    • Will the site selection allow for normal positioning of the extremity?
3. Consider the age of the patient.

Table 5-1. Characteristics of Veins and Arteries

Vein	Artery
Flow toward the heart	Flow away from the heart
Superficial vessels lie in superficial fascia; deep vessels located near arteries	Normally located deep and usually surrounded by muscle
Blood dark red	Blood bright red
Pulsations absent	Pulsations present
Valves present	Valves absent

- Infants, children, and the elderly may require sites differing from those of the adult (see Chapter 7).
4. Consider the availability and condition of the vessels.
5. Consider the following areas:
   - Is the vessel a vein or an artery? (Table 5-1)
   - Is a central or peripheral vein required? (Refer to Table 3-3 for a comparison.)
   - Can resilient vessels be palpated?
   - Is the vessel phlebotic?
   - Is the vessel located in an area that was infiltrated recently?
   - Is the vessel tortuous?
   - Is the vessel located in the upper or lower extremity?
   - Has the patient experienced injury or surgery in the area being considered?
6. Assess the size of the vessel.
   - Is the size of the vessel sufficient for delivery of the volumes of fluid required?
   - Is the size of the vessel in relationship to the size of the infusion device (vein/cannula ratio) sufficient to allow for adequate blood dilution of the infusate?
   - Is the size of the vessel in relationship to the size of the infusion device sufficient to minimize mechanical irritation between the device and the endothelial cells of the vessel wall?

General Guidelines

1. Select peripheral sites for short-term therapy, nonirritating medications, or isotonic solutions (Fig. 5-2).
2. Select central sites for long-term therapy, infusion of irritating solutions, and parenteral nutrition.
3. Avoid sites in the lower extremities, since they increase patient immobility, are more prone to thrombosis formation, and contain more valves.
4. Select the most distal site on the extremity.
5. Avoid extremities affected by injury, illness, prior surgeries (the arm on the same side as a past mastectomy), A-V shunts, or prior IV therapy.
6. Select resilient vessels.

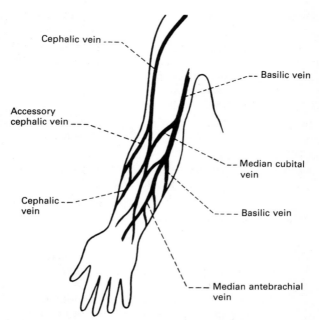

Figure 5-2. Forearm peripheral veins (Metheny N: Fluid and Electrolyte Balance, p 131. Philadelphia, JB Lippincott, 1987).

7. Avoid bifurcations and valves.
8. Avoid areas of flexion.
9. Enhance vein sighting by visualizing the site under light and observing for shadowing. This shadowing can be enhanced by wetting the area using an alcohol wipe.

Needle/Cannula Selection

The following list summarizes the recommendations for selection of infusion devices.

Patient	Situation	Device
Adult	Trauma Infusion of large amounts of fluid	14- to 18-gauge cannula 19-gauge needle
Adult	General infusion	20-gauge cannula 21-gauge needle
Adult or child	Keeping vein open Administering medications General infusion	22-gauge cannula 23-gauge needle
Infants or elderly	General infusion	24-gauge cannula 25-gauge needle
Neonates	For use in extremely small veins	27-gauge needle

Vein Dilatation Methods

1. Tourniquet
   - Place the tourniquet (rubber tubing, Velcro strap, blood pressure cuff) 4 to 6 inches above the venipuncture site.
   - Ensure that the tourniquet is not too tight by checking for the pulse after placing the tourniquet.
2. Gravity
   - Position the extremity containing the site lower

than the heart for several minutes to allow the
veins to fill.
  - Apply the tourniquet afterward.
3. Milking
  - Use a stroking or massaging motion moving from
    proximal to distal in the extremity containing the
    site.
4. Tapping
  - Gently tap over the venipuncture site with the
    tourniquet in place.
5. Fist clenching
  - Instruct the patient to open and close the fist sev-
    eral times with the tourniquet in place.
6. Warm compresses
  - Apply hot (105°F) towels to the entire extremity
    for 10 to 15 minutes prior to insertion. Do not
    apply the tourniquet until after the compress is
    removed.
7. Relaxation
  - Promote relaxation in the patient to minimize
    vasoconstriction/venous spasms caused by the
    vasovagal response to fear.
  - Visualization or mental imagery can be used to
    reduce stress (fear, anxiety, and pain) and en-
    hance relaxation (Courtemanche, 1984).
  - In addition, the nurse promotes relaxation in the
    patient by demonstrating a high level of confi-
    dence and competence and ensuring that the pa-
    tient is comfortable.

Preinsertion Local Anesthesia

Local anesthesia can be used by personnel specifically
trained for such techniques.

Purposes

Local anesthesia can be used as follows:
  - When the infusion device to be inserted is greater than
    18 gauge
  - When the patient is apprehensive

Advantages and Disadvantages

1. Perceived advantages of local anesthesia include the following:
   - Decreased pain experienced during venipuncture
   - Decreased patient apprehension
   - Decreased nurse's anxiety related to concern about causing pain
2. Perceived disadvantages of local anesthesia include the following:
   - Increased cost
   - Increased possibility of allergic reactions
   - Increased pain caused by an extra needle stick; burning
   - Increased potential for contamination/infection.

1% Lidocaine (Xylocaine)

Use of lidocaine has been controversial; some practitioners assert that the injection of normal saline produces the same advantages without some of the potential disadvantages (Wallace et al, 1983; O'Donnell, 1985; Millam, 1985; Warren, 1985). If normal saline is used, follow the same procedure of injection as outlined below, replacing the lidocaine with normal saline.

Procedure
1. Ensure that the patient is not allergic to lidocaine or related local anesthetic agents.
2. Using a tuberculin (or similar) syringe, draw up 1 ml of 1% lidocaine.
3. Put on sterile gloves.
4. Locate the venipuncture site, release the tourniquet, cleanse the site.
5. Insert the syringe needle at a 15-degree to 30-degree angle into the subcutaneous tissue.
6. After aspirating, inject a small amount of lidocaine, producing a wheal.
7. Advance the needle and inject additional amounts of lidocaine, producing a wheal each time.

8. Withdraw the needle and allow 45 to 90 seconds for the anesthetic to take effect.

Topical Anesthetic (Ethyl Chloride)

Application of a topical anesthetic is sometimes recommended, especially in the pediatric patient (Streckfuss, 1984).

Site Preparation

Shaving

Shaving produces microabrasions that may contribute to increased contamination/infection rates. It is not recommended. If hair must be removed, clipping or use of a dipilatory is advised. The use of battery-operated hair trimmers has been advocated for safe preparation of the peripheral IV site (Comella, 1986).

Cleansing of Site

The extremity of the venipuncture site should be cleansed with soap and water if necessary prior to preparing the specific site. Following cleansing, site preparation alternatives include the following:

1. 1% to 2% tincture of iodine
   - Preferred cleansing agent
   - Kills bacteria, fungi, protozoa, viruses, yeasts
   - Ensure that the patient is not allergic to iodine preparations.
   - Cleanse the venipuncture site by liberally applying the agent with a firm, circular motion (Fig. 5-3) starting at the point of venipuncture and moving in an outward circle.
   - Allow the solution to remain in contact for at least 30 seconds.
   - Remove excess iodine with 70% alcohol by lightly wiping site with sterile gauze, again using a circular, outward motion.

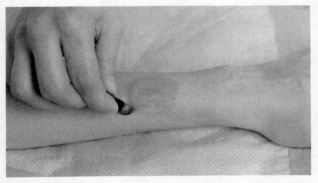

Figure 5-3. Venipuncture site is cleaned by applying a cleansing agent with a firm circular motion.

2. Povidone-iodine
    - Causes less irritation than other iodine preparations
    - Kills bacteria, fungi, protozoa, viruses, yeasts
    - Ensure that the patient is not allergic to iodine preparations.
    - Cleanse the area in the manner outlined in number 1.
    - Allow the solution to remain in contact for at least 30 seconds.
    - Do not remove the povidone-iodine since it exerts a time-release effect.
3. 70% alcohol
    - Recommended cleansing agent for patients who are allergic to iodine
    - Ineffective against tubercle bacilli, viruses, and spore-forming organisms
    - Advantages include its germicidal nature and effectiveness as a fat solvent.
    - Cleanse the area in the manner outlined above for 1 minute.
    - Repeat cleansing two additional times.

- Allow the solution to remain in contact with the skin for at least 60 seconds.

Remember: After the site is prepared, do not contaminate by touching.

Vein Entry

After rechecking the quality of the infusion device selected, complete the following steps for vein entry:

1. Attach a saline-filled syringe to the needle or cannula if applicable.
2. Reapply the tourniquet.
3. Put on sterile gloves.
4. Anchor the vein by stretching the skin 2 to 3 inches distal to the site. Pulling the skin taut reduces rolling of the vessel and eases vessel entry.
5. Insert the infusion device, bevel up, at a 20° to 30° angle in the direction of venous blood return. *Note:* A sharper angle may result in piercing of the opposite wall.
6. Use one of the following methods for vein entry:
   Direct method. Penetrate the skin at the venipuncture site and all layers of the vessel in *one* movement. This method can be used by approaching the vessel from the top or the side.
   Indirect method. In the *first* movement, penetrate the skin from the top or side slightly distal to the point of venipuncture. Then decrease the angle of the insertion device to almost parallel to the skin surface and, in a *second* movement, penetrate the vessel wall.
7. If the patient complains of severe pain, burning, tingling, or numbness, immediately remove the infusion device.
8. Observe for blood return.

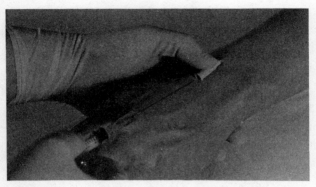

Figure 5-4. Withdraw stylet completely after the cannula has been advanced in the vein.

9. If using a steel needle and a blood return is present, advance the needle.
10. If using a cannula and a blood return is present, disengage the cannula from the stylet at least ¼ inch, advance the cannula into position; and then remove the stylet completely (Fig. 5-4).
11. If no blood return is observed, check placement of device, release tourniquet, attach to administration set, and infuse a small amount of infusate. Observe for swelling. If no swelling is observed, advance infusion device. If swelling occurs, remove infusion device.
12. Ensure proper placement and confirm unrestricted flow.
13. No more than two consecutive attempts at vein entry should occur.

Stabilization

Method of Stabilization

1. Chevron method (Fig. 5-5)
   • Using a strip of tape ¼ to ½ inch in diameter,

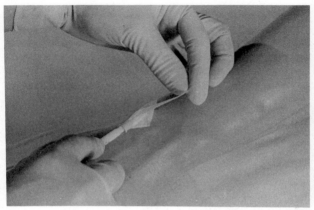

Figure 5-5. Stabilize the cannula; using the chevron method apply the tape, sticky side up, in a "V" formation just distal to the cannula shaft.

apply sticky side up in a "V" formation just distal to the cannula shaft.

- A second chevron can be applied over the first chevron.
- This method is applicable for both scalp vein and plastic cannula/catheters.

2. U method
   - Using a strip of tape ¼ to ½ inch in diameter, apply sticky side up under the hub and fold each tape tail over each corresponding wing in the U formation.
   - Use for the scalp vein needle.

3. H method
   - Place a piece of 1-inch tape vertically over each wing.
   - Place a piece of 1-inch tape horizontally over the wings forming the letter H (Fig. 5-6).
   - Use for the scalp vein needle.

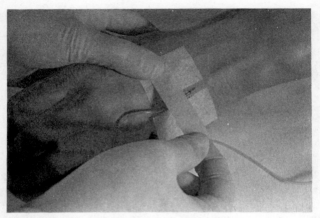

Figure 5-6. Stabilizing winged-tip needle—H method.

General Taping Tips

1. Secure the tubing to the patient's extremity by looping and taping the tubing approximately 6 inches above the venipuncture site.
2. Use the smallest amount of tape possible.
3. Do not cover the actual venipuncture site.
4. Back the tape with another piece of tape when securing the infusion device to a hairy area.
5. Use paper or nonallergic tape for those patients with sensitivity to adhesive tape.
6. Consider use of 2 to 3 inches of instant stretch bandage placed over the IV site to prevent tape from pulling away (Hunker, 1983).

Additional Considerations

1. Commercial products for anchoring the catheter hub to the skin are available.
2. Always ensure unrestricted flow after stabilizing.

3. Additional stabilization can be provided by use of armboards, contour splints, and tongue blades. The following are guidelines for the use of boards:
   - Ensure movement of fingers after armboard placement.
   - Secure with tape above and below the joint to be immobilized.
   - Secure with gauze instead of tape if appropriate.
   - Assess for adequate movement and circulation frequently.

Topical Ointments

Using ointments at the venipuncture site is controversial. Studies have failed to show a significant reduction in phlebitis rates between use and nonuse of ointments at the site (Povidone-iodine ointment, 1984). The National Intravenous Therapy Association (NITA) guidelines recommend that if topical ointment is used, an antimicrobial ointment such as povidone-iodine should be selected. The Centers for Disease Control (CDC) notes that topical polyantibiotic ointments appear to decrease infection when used for insertions requiring a cutdown and may for other insertions, but that antiseptic ointment affords little if any benefit for most insertions.

Consistent with NITA guidelines, if ointment is used, a small amount of a povidone-iodine ointment is recommended if the patient is not allergic to iodine.

Dressings

A sterile dressing should be applied to the site following complete removal of any blood or other moisture that may have accumulated.

Types

1. Gauze dressings
   - Place over the venipuncture site and secure well with tape.

Table 5-2. Examples of
Transparent Dressing

Tape	Manufacturer
Bioclusive	Johnson & Johnson
Ensure	Deseret
Opraflex	Lehmann
Op-Site	Smith & Nephew
Polyskin	Kendall
Tegaderm	3-M
Uniflex	United
Visulin	Wurhilin

- Label the dressing tape. Include type, length, and gauge of infusion device; date and time of insertion; and initials of the person inserting the device.
2. Transparent dressings
   - Adhesive-coated, semipermeable film is available from numerous manufacturers (Table 5-2).
   - Advantages of this type of dressing include continuous observation of the site, effective protection against infection, and cost-effectiveness (Freeman and Boyer, 1982; Jones et al, 1982, Peck, 1985).

Application Guidelines

1. After insertion of the device, remove any excess moisture from the skin surface.
2. Secure the cannula hub with a ½-inch-wide strip of nonallergic tape.
3. Center the transparent dressing over the cannula and cover up to, but not over, the cannula–tubing connection. This will allow for tubing changes without necessarily dressing changes.
4. Ensure a thorough seal of the dressing around the hub area by pressing on both sides of the hub.
5. Smooth the dressing outward as the rest of the paper backing is removed.
6. Write on a provided label or piece of tape the following:

- Type, length of gauge of infusion device
- Date and time of insertion
- Initials of person inserting the device

7. Place the label on the corner of the dressing; do not cover the insertion site.

Note: Use of small Band-Aids is not recommended since they do not adequately cover and protect the site and surrounding area.

Flow Rate

Formula for Calculating the Flow Rate Using Macrodrip Tubing

$$\text{gtt/min} = \frac{\text{gtt/ml of adm. set}}{60 \text{ min}}$$

$$\times \text{ total hourly volume (ml)}$$

1. Count the drops over 1 minute.
2. Set the flow clamp.
3. Recheck the rate at ½-hour intervals for 1 hour.

Refer to Chapter 4 to review the numerous factors that influence and change the flow rate.

Calculation of Flow Rate Using Microdrip Tubing

1. For all microdrip tubing, the number of drops per minute equals the number of milliliters per hour (Jones and Thaw, 1985).
2. To calculate number of milliliters to be delivered per minute:

$$\text{ml/min} = \frac{\text{number of ml/hr}}{60}$$

3. To calculate number of drops per minute:

$$\text{gtts/min} = (\text{ml/min}) \times 60 \text{ gtt/ml}$$

KVO-TKO Rates

The "keep vein open" (TKO, KVO, KO) order is defined differently depending on clinical agency, clinical area, physician, and patient condition, age, and history. It can mean administering 0.6 ml/hr to 100 ml/hr. It is recommended that institutional policy be developed to indicate a prescribed maximum volume infusion per patient situation (Friedman, 1982).

Electronic Flow Devices

If the electronic flow devices—controllers or pumps—are to be used, follow the specific instructions accompanying each device. (See Chapter 3 to review characteristics of these devices.)

Charting

The patient's record should document the following information regarding insertion:

1. Type, size, and gauge of infusion device
2. Type of infusion set used
3. Type, amount, and number of infusate container, including all additives
4. Site of venipuncture
5. Flow rate
6. Type of controller/pump used, if applicable
7. Type of filter used, if applicable
8. Patient's tolerance of insertion procedure
9. Observations of site
10. Use of any ancillary devices (*i.e.*, armboard)
11. Overall condition of patient
12. Reasons for discontinuing previous infusion device, if applicable
13. Unsuccessful insertion attempts, including a complete description of what happened and the status of the patient's venous system
14. Name and credentials of person initiating the therapy

Bibliography

Burrows C: Take a step toward making better I.V. needle selections. Nursing84 14:32–33, 1984

Chrystal C: Selecting an I.V. tubing system. Infect Control 6(9):384, 1985

Comella M: Hair trimmers safely prep peripheral I.V. site. NITA Update 7(6):4, 1986

Courtemanche J: Imagery enhances venipuncture. NITA 7:30, 1984

Darby T, Ausman R: Particulate matter in polyvinyl chloride intravenous bags. N Engl J Med 290:579, 1974

Freeman P, Boyer J: How to get the most out of OP-SITE. RN 45(1):37–39, 1982

Friedman F: KVO's: How fast is fast enough? RN 45(9):69–74, 1982

Handwashing for nurses. NITA Update 7(2):7, 1986

Hospital infection control. Handwashing Agents. NITA Update 6(2):2, 1985

Hunker M: I.V. taping tip. NITA Update 4(1):6, 1983

Infection traced to false fingernails. NITA Updated 6(6):6, 1985

Jones B, Briggs C, Norton D: I.V. dressing. Nursing82 12:70–73, 1982

Jones M, Thaw P: Tips for calculating I.V. rates in an emergency. RN 48:44, 1985

Larson EB, Dowell S, Scott D: Inadequate medical order writing and delivery: A cause of unnecessary hospital costs. QRB 10(11):353, 1984

Maki D, Band J: A comparative study of polyantibiotic and iodophor ointment in prevention of vascular catheter-related infection. Am J Med 76:739, 1981

Metheny N: Fluid and Electrolyte Balance, p 131. Philadelphia, JB Lippincott, 1987

Millam D: Using a local anesthetic for I.V. insertion. Nurs Life 5:52–53, 1985

Nitroglycerin ointment as an aid to venipuncture. NITA Update 4(3):4, 1983

O'Donnell J: Lidocaine use for placing I.V. cannulas. NITA 8:69, 1985

Paduano M: Calculate IV drip rates—with ease. RN 47:59–60, 1984

Pauley S: Nitro vein dilation. NITA Update 6(2):5, 1985

Peck N: Perfecting your I.V. therapy techniques, Part I. Nursing85 15:38–43, 1985

Peck N: Perfecting your I.V. therapy techniques, Part III. Nursing85 15:32–35, 1985

Povidone-iodine ointment with transparent dressings. NITA Update 5:3, 1984

Streckfuss B: Topical anesthetics for children? NITA Update 4:3, 1984

Wallace A, Whitcomb V, Kohler S: Use of lidocaine as a local anesthetic. NITA Update 4(5):4, 1983

Warren J: Using a local anesthetic for I.V. insertion. Nursing Life 5:52–53, Jan/Feb 1985

6 ▷ Maintaining and Discontinuing Intravenous Therapy

Key Points

1. Maintaining effective IV therapy:
   - Solution
   - Tubing
   - Needle/cannula/catheter
   - Dressings/site assessment
   - Nursing observations
   - Guidelines for nursing interventions
   - Patient education
   - Charting
2. Discontinuing therapy

Maintaining Effective IV Therapy

Maintaining effective IV therapy is dependent on the following:

Solution

The same infusate container should hang for no longer than 24 hours. Beyond this length of time, microbial growth can occur.

Tubing

1. Although some research indicates that use of the same tubing is safe for up to 4 days (Josephson et al, 1985), it is recommended that tubing be changed every 48 hours (McGowan, 1980; Reilly, 1985; Turco, 1980).

2. Tubing changes every 24 hours may be indicated if numerous medications or parenteral nutrition are being infused or if intermittent devices are being used. These situations increase demands on the filter.
3. Change the tubing every 24 hours if the system is being entered or interrupted more than a few times in the 48-hour interval (Chrystal, 1985).
4. Maintain correct labeling that documents the date, time, and initials of the professional hanging the tubing.
5. Ensure that all connections are tight and secure.

Needle/Cannula/Catheter

1. It is recommended that the peripheral needle or cannula be changed every 48 to 72 hours. Central lines operate under different guidelines. (See Chapter 11 for details.)
2. Use of a site rotation diagram can facilitate site selection. The diagram should include the available vessels of the extremity. As each site is used, the diagram is marked to indicate the site and date used.

Dressings/Site Assessment

1. Traditional gauze dressings
   - Change every 24 to 48 hours
   - Assess site.
   - Cleanse area with antiseptic.
   - Use an antimicrobial ointment if policy indicates.
2. Transparent dressings
   - Change when the site is rotated.
   - Assess the site every 8 hours.
3. Sites are assessed for the following:
   - Redness
   - Edema
   - Drainage
   - Leakage

Nursing Observations

1. General response of the patient to IV therapy as it relates to the goal(s) of therapy
2. Discomfort of patient
3. Equipment functioning
4. Signs and symptoms of local and septicemic complications (see Chapters 8 and 9)
5. Rate maintenance. At 1- to 2-hour intervals, at a minimum, note the following:
   - The fluid level in the infusate container
   - The rate of flow. Note that less than 15% of the flow-rate observations recorded in a recent study were within the range of ±10% of the desired drip rate and only 21% were over ±20% accurate (Crass and Vance, 1985).
   - The integrity of the tubing and connections
   - The condition of the site
6. Infused volume. Record volume infused at regular intervals, and when reading fluid levels, read at eye level. When recording volume infused from plastic bags note that the number at each mark identifies the amount of fluid infused (*e.g.,* "1" means 100 ml has been infused).

Guidelines for Nursing Interventions

1. Never measure the blood pressure in the extremity with the venipuncture site.
2. Keep the flow clamp above the level of the heart.
3. If the rate slows, attempt to correct as follows:
   - Increase the height of the infusate container.
   - Increase the flow clamp.
   - *Never* lower the container below the venipuncture site to elicit a blood return. Allowing the blood to back up and remain in the administration tubing creates a medium for bacterial growth.
   - *Never* insert a needle for an airway.
4. Check for vein patency, indicated by one or more of the following:

- Blood return by squeezing the flashball
- Freely running solution
- No discomfort or burning at the site
- No leakage of fluid around the site

5. Avoid irrigating the infusion device.
   - Irrigating an established clot is rarely successful; if the clot has existed less than 15 minutes it can sometimes be irrigated.
   - If irrigation is indicated and in accordance with institutional policy, it is recommended that a tuberculin-size syringe containing normal saline be used at the port closest to the cannula and the strictest aseptic technique be maintained. The administration tubing is kinked as the normal saline is infused (Kaminski and Pluta, 1978).

6. Use strict aseptic techniques. *Remember:* manipulation and touch contamination are major causes of complications. Every manipulation, entrance, and component of the infusion system increases the chance of development of complications and contamination rates.

7. If the IV tubing becomes disconnected, replace with a new cannula and tubing. If contamination of fluid is suspected, the infusate container should also be replaced.

8. If an air bubble is found in the tubing, it can sometimes be removed by aspirating the fluid in the tubing from the port just distal to the bubble, using a sterile needle attached to a sterile syringe. However, changing the tubing is recommended.

Patient Education

Instruct the patient in the following:

1. Do not kink or compress the IV tubing
2. When moving the extremity with the venipuncture site, move the whole extremity as a unit.
3. Use the extremity without the infusion for routine activities.

4. Do not lie on the IV.
5. Use the armboard.
6. Do not adjust the flow clamp, IV pole, and so forth.
7. When walking, do the following:
   - Call the nurse for help.
   - Do not pull on IV tubing.
   - Use the IV pole.
   - Keep the IV arm at waist level.
8. Call the nurse in the following situations:
   - If the container is almost empty
   - If pain, burning, redness, or swelling is experienced
   - If the site or lines are wet or if blood is present
   - If the site is bumped

Note: Patients, particularly those with fragile veins and in need of frequent IV therapy, may be instructed to build up their veins through hand exercises, such as squeezing a small rubber ball (Raising veins, 1987).

Charting

1. Document the following:
   - Condition of the tubing
   - Site care
   - Dressing changes
   - Condition of the site
   - Rotation of sites
   - Patient education
2. Flow sheets for recording IV procedures are helpful and should include the following components (Schatzel, 1985):
   - Date and time
   - Initials
   - Start, restart
   - Cannula type, gauge, length
   - Cannula site
   - Heparin lock
   - Reason for site change (*e.g.,* phlebitis, pulled out, leaking, occluded, hospital policy)

- Purpose of site (*e.g.,* primary, piggyback, push medications, blood)
- Date and initials for IV rounds
- Heparinization
- Dressing change

Discontinuing Therapy

1. Review the physician's order.
2. Provide an explanation to the patient.
3. Remove the armboard, tape, and dressing.
4. Observe the site.
5. Close the flow clamp.
6. Lay a sterile gauze over the site. *Do not apply pressure.*
7. Put on sterile gloves.
8. Withdraw the needle/cannula, keeping the hub parallel with the skin surface. *Do not lift up on the hub.*
9. Apply pressure to the site.
10. Observe and measure, if indicated, the length of the needle, cannula, or catheter.
11. Culture the needle, cannula, or catheter only if a cannula-related infection is suspected. It is not recommended that needles or cannulas be routinely cultured.
12. Tape a sterile dressing (pressure dressing) in place.
13. Complete documentation should include the type, size, and gauge of the infusion device removed, why removed, the condition of the site and infusion device, patient response, type of dressing applied, date, time, and signature.

Bibliography

Byers P: Comparison of application factors among three brands of transparent semi-permeable films for peripheral IVs. NITA 8:315, 1985

Byers P, Burke E, and Overstake S: Reading the amount of fluid in polyvinyl chloride I.V. bags. NITA 9(6):484, 1986

Chrystal C: Selecting an I.V. tubing system. Infect Control 6(9):384, 1985

Crass R, Vance J: In-view accuracy of gravity-flow I.V. infusion systems. Am J Hosp Pharm 42:328, 1985

Fallout. Nursing86 16:9, 1986

Haessler RM: Transparent I.V. dressings, vs. traditional dressings. NITA 6:169, 1983

Josephson A, Gombert M, Sierra M et al: The relationship between intravenous fluid contamination and the frequency of tubing replacement. Infect Control 6(9):367, 1985

Kaminski K: Irrigation. Am J Intravenous Ther Clin Nutr 5:23, 1978

Lawson M: Comparison of transparent dressing to paper tape dressing over the central venous catheter site. NITA 9:40, 1986

McGowan JE: How often should administration tubing be changed in I.V. therapy? Am J Intravenous Ther Clin Nutr 7:19, 1980

Nicola M, DeChairo D: A transparent polyurethane membrane used as an I.V. dressing. NITA 7:139, 1984

Peck N: Perfecting your IV therapy techniques, part III. Nursing 85 15:32–35, 1985

Popousky M, Ilstrup D: Randomized clinical trial of transparent polyurethane I.V. dressings. NITA 9:107, 1986

Raising veins. Nursing87 17:9, 1987

Reilly K: Tubing changes. NITA Update 6(1):5, 1985

Schatzel J: I.V. therapy record sheet. NITA 8(3):242, 1985

Turco S: 24 or 48 hour administration set change? Am J Intravenous Ther Clin Nutr 7:11, 1980

7 ▷ Special Infusion Situations: Geriatric Patients, Pediatric Patients, Heparin Locks

Key Points

1. Geriatric patients
   - Physiological changes in aging
   - Specific nursing interventions
2. Pediatric patients
   - Psychological characteristics of the child
   - Physical characteristics of the child
   - Nursing interventions for initiating IV therapy in the pediatric patient
3. Heparin locks
   - Types
   - Advantages
   - Disadvantages
   - Uses
   - Insertion
   - Maintenance

Geriatric Patients

Physiological Changes in Aging

Unique changes and needs in the elderly patient have implications for delivery of IV therapy. The following physiological changes influence initiating and maintaining therapy in the elderly patient:

1. Increased density and amount of collagen fibers in the vessel walls
2. Decreased elasticity of the vessel wall

3. Progressive straightening, fraying, splitting, and fragmenting of elastic fibers in the vessel walls
4. Decreased distensibility of vessels
5. Increased peripheral resistance
6. Possible increase in the adhesiveness of platelets
7. Increased difficulty in hearing
8. Possible increase in confusion

Specific Nursing Interventions

1. Infusion device. Scalp vein needles are the preferred infusion device for the following reasons:
   - They are more maneuverable.
   - The wing construction decreases the potential for contamination.
   - The wings lie flat against the skin, providing a more fixed, stable device.
   - They are less thrombogenic.
   - Success in using 22-gauge infusion devices has been noted (Ingalls, 1984).
2. Vein selection
   Differentiate between vein wall quality by noting the following:
   - Sclerosed veins are resistant to pressure.
   - Sturdy veins are firm to the touch and resilient to pressure.
   - Weak-walled (fragile) veins are soft to the touch and lack elasticity.
3. Vein dilatation
   A Velcro tourniquet is preferred over the elastic because the pressure is displaced over a broader area, decreasing the possibility of damage to fragile vessels. It also constricts blood flow in a more uniform manner. However, a tourniquet may not be required.
4. Vein puncture
   - Avoid rolling or fragile veins, if possible.
   - If rolling veins are used, consider the following:
     Use countertension to stabilize the vessel.

> Enter the vein as close to the venipuncture site as possible.
>
> Thread the needle as far as possible; by putting the entire needle in the vessel, stabilization is promoted.
>
> • Note: If veins are fragile, the procedure is as follows:
>
> Apply heat through hot compresses prior to venipuncture.
>
> Use a small-gauge needle (*e.g.*, 23 gauge).
>
> Enter the vessel slowly.

5. Stabilization

   Use of a contour splint, preferable to the conventional armboard, allows the arm to lie in a natural, comfortable manner.

6. Education needs

   Attention to the patient's mental status, level of hearing, and visual and tactile deficits is especially important.

7. Administration of additives
   • Absorption may be erratic.
   • Distribution of medications may be altered by the fat and protein tissue.
   • Metabolism may be slowed or incomplete.
   • Excretion may be slowed or inefficient.

Pediatric Patients

The pediatric patient is not only smaller, but also different from the adult. General characteristics of the pediatric patient have ramifications for IV therapy.

Psychological Characteristics of the Child

Be aware of their concerns, such as the following:

1. Fear of body injury, pain
2. Fear of separation from trusted significant others
3. Fear of moving from a familiar environment
4. Fear of the strange and unknown

5. Anxiety related to uncertainty about limits of behavior
6. Fear related to loss of control, autonomy, independence, competence, and self-esteem
7. Decreased ability to understand and cooperate

Implications for nursing interventions should include the following:

1. Acknowledge the fears and anxieties.
2. Provide emotional support appropriate to age.
3. Allow the child choices whenever possible.
4. Let the child know that the fears are all right and that crying is OK.
5. Encourage significant others to stay with the child.
6. Prepare significant others for the procedure by providing support, encouragement, and information.
7. Provide support before, during, *and* after the procedure by giving praise, holding, and cuddling.
8. Let the child act or play out the fears.
9. Provide educational materials appropriate to the child's age.

Physical Characteristics of the Child

1. Children have a high water content in the body.
2. Greater water turnover occurs in the child due to a greater surface area, greater insensible loss, higher metabolic rate, and decreased ability to concentrate urine due to immature kidneys.
3. Children are more susceptible to dehydration.

Assessment for dehydration should include the following:

1. Weight loss
2. Decreased blood pressure
3. Poor skin turgor
4. Dry mucous membranes
5. Increased pulse
6. Increased temperature

7. Decreased central nervous system activity
8. Increased urine specific gravity
9. Decreased urine output
10. Lack of tear formation
11. Thirst
12. Lethargy
13. Sunken eyeballs
14. Sunken anterior fontanelle
15. High-pitched cry

Nursing Interventions for Initiating IV Therapy in the Pediatric Patient

The following guidelines represent nursing interventions specific for the pediatric patient that deviate from the guidelines outlined in Chapter 5 for initiating IV therapy.

1. Infusate
   · Use a container of 250 ml or less.
2. Administration set
   · Use a volume control set.
   · Use a controller/pump as appropriate.

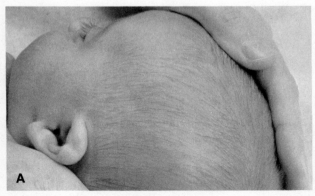

Figure 7-1. Infusion sites for an infant. *A:* Scalp vein. *B:* Hand. *C:* Ankle.

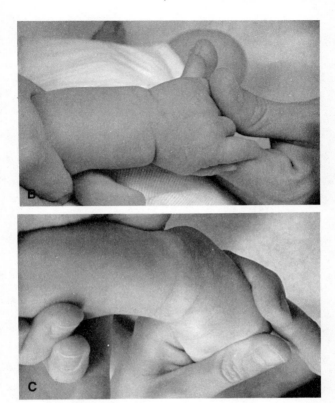

Figure 7-1.   (Continued)

3. Venipuncture site (Fig. 7-1).
   - The scalp vessels and umbilical site are used for the newborn, neonate, and infant.
   - The dorsal foot is recommended for the toddler.
   - The site that is least vulnerable to infiltration is preferred.
   - The site that requires the least amount of restraints is preferred.

- Peripheral sites are preferred for administering all infusate except the extremely hypertonic.
- Peripheral sites allow more mobility, involve less risk, and are less disfiguring.

4. Infusion device
- Scalp vein needles are preferred because they are less painful on insertion, are less injurious to vessels, and decrease the potential for seeding of bacteria.
- It is recommended that a 23 to 25 gauge be used for the neonate, 21 to 23 gauge for the infant/toddler, 19 to 23 gauge for the school-age child, and 19 to 21 gauge for an adolescent (Matyskiela, 1984).
- Over-the-needle cannulas are recommended for long-term therapy or administration of antibiotics or parenteral nutrition. They are recommended when a peripheral site cannot be maintained for 72 hours or when the client has poor venous access. They need be changed only every 2 weeks (Stephens and Rans, 1987). Recommended sizes include 24 gauge for the neonate, 20 to 24 gauge for the infant/toddler, 18 to 24 gauge for the school-age child, and 16 to 22 gauge for an adolescent (Matyskiela, 1984).

5. Venipuncture
- Perform the procedure in a room separate from the child's room.
- Always use a saline-filled syringe with the scalp vein infusion device.
- Use mummy and clove-hitch restraints as needed.
- Omit tourniquet use if possible.
- Use direct entry approach. Flush the needle immediately on entry into the vessel.
- Decrease discomfort by using a topical anesthetic, controlled breathing, and distraction.

6. Stabilization
- Tongue blades may be useful as a splint.
- One half of a paper cup is not recommended to

cover the infusion site on the scalp (Jarmen, 1985); use only stabilization devices specifically designed for IV therapy use.

7. Rotation of sites is not routinely done on the pediatric patient.

Heparin Locks

A heparin lock is an infusion device capped by a resealable latex diaphragm that allows for intermittent IV administration by keeping the vein open (KVO) between administrations. (See Chapter 3 for figures.)

Types

1. An existing IV device that can be adapted by adding a resealable post
2. A standard scalp vein (winged) heparin lock needle

Advantages

1. Provide continuous access to the vein
2. Allow more flexibility/mobility, safety, and comfort for the patient
3. Allow for infusion of a reduced fluid volume
4. Eliminate KVO bottles/bags
5. Are available for collection of blood samples
6. Allow medication administration outside hospital
7. Cost less than a continuous infusion
8. Are more convenient for nursing personnel since monitoring of continuous flow is not required
9. Yield lower phlebitis rates
10. Cause less vein irritation

Disadvantages

1. Occlusion can occur, as evidenced by no flow or no blood return.
2. Some drugs are incompatible with heparin.
3. Use of a large-bore needle for adding medication may damage the diaphragm.

4. Speed shock may occur if a medication is administered too rapidly.
5. A drug may be administered IV push inadvertently when it should have been diluted first.

Uses

1. Intermittent IV medications
2. Venous access for emergency medications
3. Venous access for blood samples

Insertion

1. Refer to Chapter 5 for preparation of the patient and selection and preparation of equipment.
2. Prior to insertion of the heparin lock, wipe the injection port with alcohol and instill 1 ml of normal saline using a syringe.
3. Leave the syringe attached to the port.
4. Put on sterile gloves.
5. Insert the heparin lock as outlined in Chapter 5.
6. Ensure patency and remove the syringe.
7. Complete stabilization, dressings, and charting as outlined in Chapter 5.
8. Heparinize the lock by injecting 0.2 ml to 0.5 ml of heparin (1 : 10 to 1 : 100 or 1 : 1000 units) using a 22- or 25-gauge needle.

Maintaining the Heparin Lock

Maintaining vein patency can be accomplished by two methods:

1. Intermittent heparin flush
   · Heparinize with 0.2 ml to 0.5 ml of heparin after every dosage of medication, or at least every 8 hours, using a 22- or 25-gauge needle.
   · If administering a medication, first flush with 2 ml normal saline, administer medication, flush again with 2 ml normal saline, and then heparinize the lock as previously outlined (Farrell, 1984).

- Common medications incompatible with heparin include morphine, demerol, atropine, diazepam, furosemide (Lasix), gentamicin, and tobramycin.
2. Intermittent saline flush
   - Instead of the heparin flush, some institutions have used saline flushes with equal success in maintaining vessel patency (Harrigan, 1985).
   - The lock is irrigated with 2 ml sodium chloride at least every 12 hours.
3. A flush is used before and after the administration of medications.
4. Rotation of heparin lock sites should occur every 48 to 72 hours.
5. Discontinuing heparin locks follows the procedure outlined in Chapter 6.

Bibliography

Alfano G: The older adult and drug therapy. Geriatric Nurs 3:28–30, 1982

Barfoot K: Home care of the child receiving nutritional support. NITA 9(3):226, 1986

Briggs L, Beyda D: Giving pediatric code drugs. Nursing86 16:56–57, July 1986

Crass R, Vance J: In-vivo accuracy of gravity-flow I.V. infusion systems. Am J Hosp Pharm 42:328, 1985

Dolby B: 1983. Caution: Abused veins, handle with care. NITA 6(2):95, 1983

Farrell J: 1984. Tips for avoiding intravenous medication errors. Parenterals 2(6):1, 1984

Frey A: Pediatric dosage calculations. NITA 8(5):373, 1985

Gardner C: INT devices. NITA Update 5(4):7, 1984

Harrigan CA: Intermittent I.V. therapy without heparin: A study. NITA 8:519, 1985

Ingalls M: 22-Gauge catheters. NITA Update 5(4):7, 1984

Jarmen C: Vein trauma—its complications and prevention. Intravenous Ther News 12(7):4, 1985

Koren G: Improved technique for intravenous drug delivery in children. Am J Intravenous Ther Clin Nutr 9:33, 1983

Leff R: Intravenous administration of medications to the pediatric patient. NITA 6(4):255, 1983

Matyskiela A: Pediatric I.V. devices. Parenterals 2:3, 1984

Nahata M: Methods of intravenous drug infusion in pediatric patients. Am J Intravenous Ther Clin Nutr 11(5):6, 1984

Oelerich W, Dombrowski J: Mini I.V. patients in maximum precautions. RN 44:43–47, 1981

Peck N: Perfecting I.V. therapy techniques, Part II. Nursing85 15:48–51, 1985

Piercy S: Children on long-term I.V. therapy. Nursing81 11:66–69, 1981

Schustek M: A cost-effective approach to PRN service maintenance. NITA 7(6):527, 1984

Stephens B, Rans M: Use of intracaths in pediatric intravenous therapy. NITA Update 8(1):4, 1987

Streckfuss B: Communicating with pediatric patients. NITA 7(2):94, 1984

Streckfuss B: Pediatric I.V. care. NITA 8(1):75, 1985

Teitall B: Considerations for neonatal I.V. therapy. NITA 7(6):521, 1984

Turco S: Heparin locks. Am J Intravenous Ther Clin Nutr 10:9–12, 1983

Waidley E: Show and tell—preparing children for invasive procedures. AJN 85:811–812, 1985

Zerwekh J: The dehydration question. Nursing83 13:47–51, 1983

Unit III

Complications of Intravenous Therapy

8 ▷ Local Complications

The practitioner must be fully alert to the hazards that accompany IV therapy. With the continuous introduction of new equipment, infusates, medications, and numerous devices, complications still assume a sometimes insignificant level of attention. Only when the practitioner fully understands all complications, their causes and avenues for prevention, can the safest, most effective care be ensured. Discussion of each type of localized complication, including causes, assessment/evaluation, and nursing interventions for the treatment or prevention of the complication, follows.

Vein Irritation, Phlebitis, Thrombosis, Thrombophlebitis

Vein irritation, phlebitis and postinfusion phlebitis, thrombosis, and thrombophlebitis are interrelated; they are all advanced stages of the same phenomenon. Understanding normal vein structure as well as anatomical and physiological changes that occur in response to irritation clarifies this interrelationship.

Vein Physiology

The vein wall consists of three major layers:

1. *Tunica intima*. The innermost, one-cell-thick layer composed of endothelial cells
2. *Tunica media*. The middle layer containing collagen, which when exposed to blood facilitates the clotting process, possibly resulting in thrombus formation
3. *Tunica adventitia*. The outermost muscle layer

Vein Irritation Events

Early irritation of the vein wall creates mild changes including swelling of the endothelial cells and infiltration of polymorphonuclear leukocytes into the tunica media. If the irritation continues, moderate vessel changes occur including progressive cellular destruction of the tunica intima, edema of the tunica media, and early changes in the muscle cells of the tunica adventitia. Severe vein changes then occur if the irritation persists. These include destruction of the endothelium, hemorrhages and necrosis of the vein wall, and the possible development of thrombi (Ghidyal et al, 1975).

Causes of Vein Irritation

Causes of vein irritation, phlebitis, thrombus formation, and thrombophlebitis are summarized in Tables 8-1 to 8-3.

Table 8-1. Chemical Causes of Vein Irritation, Phlebitis, Thrombosis, and Thrombophlebitis

Causes	Comment/Example
Plastic cannula/catheter material	Especially polyvinyl chloride
	Phlebitis 3× more frequent with use of plastic cannula vs. needle
Plasticizers from infusate container	Leaching of plasticizers
Solution pH	pH greater than 11.0 and less than 4.3 are most irritating
	Acidic solutions become more acidic during sterilization
Solution osmolality	Hypertonic solutions (over 320 mOsm)
Type of medication	Antibiotics, chemotherapeutic drugs (vesicants: nitrogen mustard, methotrexate, [Velban], vincristine [Oncovin], vinblastine doxorubicin [Adriamycin], daunomycin, actinomycin D, mithramycin), potassium chloride, diazepam (Valium)
Method of medication administration	Too fast administration of medication decreases the ability of venous blood to naturally dilute infusate.
	Use of a large-gauge needle/cannula decreases blood's ability to dilute infusate.

Table 8-2. Mechanical Causes of Vein Irritation, Phlebitis, Thrombosis, and Thrombophlebitis

Causes	Comment/Example
Gauge of cannula/needle	
Length of cannula/needle	
Cannula/vein ratio	
Position of cannula tip	
Location of infusion site	Lower extremities more vulnerable
Movement	More movement increases phlebitis
Duration	Longer duration increases phlebitis
Particulate matter in needle/cannula, tubing, additional equipment, infusate	
Trauma of insertion	Cannula insertion more traumatizing than insertion of needle
Trauma of discontinuing the IV	

Assessment

The incidence of complications may range from 3.5% to 70% (Carlson, 1985). Assessment is, therefore, critical in minimizing and preventing such complications. Clinical signs include the following:

1. Slow IV flow rate
   (This may be the first warning sign of vein irritation.)
2. Tenderness above insertion site
3. Redness at site
4. Warmth at site
5. Possibly edema
6. Possibly pain
7. Fever

Table 8-3. Biologic Causes of Vein Irritation, Phlebitis, Thrombosis, and Thrombophlebitis

Causes	Comment/Example
Solution container	Cracked/pinholes
	Expired date
	Touch contamination especially in spiking plastic containers
Solution type	Solution hanging longer than 24 hours has greater contamination rate
Air contamination	Inrush of unfiltered air when opening glass container
	Use of unfiltered needle when preparing admixtures
Contamination during admixture	Palming of admixture syringe
	Contamination of vial tops
Catheter colonization	
Stopcocks	
Shaving	Shaving produces microabrasions
Surface bacteria movement	Skin flora enter insertion site and can ascend the infusion system as high as 5 feet against flow
Manipulations of the system/components	

Note: Prompt assessment for these signs is essential; they can indicate that the patient may be predisposed to sepsis and embolism and may cause considerable discomfort.

A specific pattern may be observed in the development of phlebitis. Initially no tenderness or discoloration is present. Within a short period, usually less than 8 hours, discoloration and tenderness develop. Next, pain may be experienced at the site. Within 8 to 16 hours additional signs may occur, including increased temperature at the infusion site, increase in body temperature by one degree, and presence of a palpable cord induration. After 16 hours, all signs continue to be present except that the skin temperature at the site may decrease. Finally, between 24 and 32 hours, the body temperature may again increase slightly (Jones and Koldjeski, 1984; Maddox et al, 1977; Turco, 1981).

Nursing Interventions to Minimize Damage

1. Discontinue the IV immediately upon evidence of vein irritation.
2. Apply warm/cold packs as ordered.

Nursing Interventions to Minimize Chemical Irritation

1. Use fresh solutions.
2. Use steel needles whenever feasible (Williams et al, 1982).
3. Use Teflon cannulas whenever possible, as this may lower the incidence of phlebitis (Tulley et al, 1981; Williams et al, 1982).
4. Use large veins for hyperosmolar (over 320 mOsm) solutions.
5. Use large veins for solutions having pH values greater than 11 or less than 4.3.
6. Provide a sound vein/cannula ratio when selecting infusion vessels and equipment.
7. Administer IV medications at as fast a rate as safety of volume and effects of medication allow.
8. Use a smaller-gauge needle for medication infusion.
9. Place the IV bag in a horizontal position when adding potassium chloride (to avoid layering of the medication), squeeze bag, and mix well before administration.
10. Whenever possible, follow infusion of hypertonic solution with an isotonic one to wash irritants away.

Nursing Interventions to Minimize Mechanical Irritation

1. Use a sound vein/cannula ratio.
2. Maintain stabilization of the needle or cannula.
3. Avoid applying excessive pressure when palpating the site.
4. Avoid use of the lower extremities.
5. Minimize trauma of insertion.
6. Limit duration of site to 24 to 48 hours; do not exceed 72 hours.
7. Minimize trauma when discontinuing the IV.
8. Minimize particulate matter infusion:
   - Use steel needles when possible.
   - Use only the equipment and amount of tubing that is absolutely essential.
   - Avoid excessive juggling and shaking of infusate containers.
   - Use filter needles for administration of admixtures, unless contraindicated (Silverman, 1985).

Nursing Interventions to Minimize Biologic Contamination

1. Inspect infusate container for cracks, pinholes, and discoloration.
2. Check expiration date of all infusates.
3. Do not infuse any solution that has been open for more than 24 hours (Amonsen and Gren, 1978).
4. Avoid palming of the syringe plunger (*i.e.,* touching the interior components of the syringe during filling).
5. Avoid use of multidose vials.
6. Avoid use of stopcocks.
7. Avoid shaving the IV site.
8. Stabilize cannula/needle to minimize movement of surface bacteria.
9. Follow procedures meticulously.
10. Minimize manipulation of the IV system.
11. Change the catheter/cannula every 48 to 72 hours to

minimize the possibility of colonization with microorganisms.

12. Use an antibacterial ointment at the site, if indicated.
13. Meticulously prepare the site.
14. Perform handwashing for at least 15 seconds.
15. *Use strict aseptic technique.*

Implementing these precautions can reduce the incidence of vein irritation to as low as 5% (Chrystal, 1985).

Suppurative Thrombophlebitis

Suppurative thrombophlebitis occurs when an infected vein develops a pocket of pus. If the purulent material moves through the circulatory system, septicemia results. Initially thrombophlebitis is caused by chemical and mechanical irritation and biologic contamination.

Assessment

Assessment of suppurative thrombophlebitis is difficult; there is generally an absence of local signs of infection or inflammation. However, three signs are to be evaluated.

1. Fever
2. Positive blood culture
3. Positive catheter tip culture

Nursing Interventions

Treatment usually involves surgical excision. The nurse's role is primarily one of assessment and prevention.

1. Constant observation and absolute adherence to aseptic techniques are musts.
2. All prevention interventions for vein irritation should be followed.
3. Patients at risk include those on immunosuppressive therapy and those having cancer and burns.

Remember: removal of the cannula/catheter does *not* make the infection disappear. The first signs of septicemia may appear 2 to 10 days after the cannula is removed.

Infiltration and Extravasation

Infiltration is the accumulation of fluid in the tissue occurring when the needle or cannula has been pulled partially or totally out of the vein. *Extravasation* is the leakage of fluid or blood from a vessel while the needle/cannula is still in place. Both complications can be minor discomforts if the fluid is isotonic or nonirritating. They can cause major irritation and tissue destruction, however, if a large amount of hypertonic fluid is involved. The incidence ranges from 1% to 11%.

Causes

1. Movement of needle/cannula
2. Unsecured needle/cannula
3. Weakened vessel wall related to vein irritation
4. Administering solution in too large amounts too fast

Assessment

Observe for the following clinical signs:

1. Pain, burning, itching, or unusual sensation
2. Slow or no infusion rate
3. No blood return observed when tubing is pinched
4. Immediate swelling or redness at the insertion site or any area proximal to the site. Compare limb size for evaluation.
5. Wet dressing
6. Hardness at site
7. Site cool to touch
8. Darkened skin within 24 hours due to tissue injury and progress to tissue destruction

Nursing Interventions

Nursing treatments are as follows:

1. Stop the IV immediately.
2. Closely observe the wound.

3. Place ice packs at the site for 15 to 20 minutes every 4 to 6 hours; continue for 72 hours (Nurse Drug Alert, 1985).
4. Elevate the limb.
5. Withdraw 4 ml to 5 ml of blood and administer hydrocortisone to decrease inflammation, if ordered by physician.
6. Administer a local anesthetic to decrease pain, if ordered by physician.
7. Administer appropriate antidotes as indicated. (Refer to Chapter 14 for a discussion of antidotes related to chemotherapeutic medications.)

Preventive nursing interventions are as follows:

1. Select the appropriate type and size of cannula/needle.
2. Stabilize the IV adequately.
3. Check the IV site frequently.
4. Administer fluid consistent with venous capacity.
5. Provide patient education regarding care of site and signs of infiltration/extravasation.

Cellulitis

Cellulitis is a diffuse inflammatory response within the tissue. It is caused by infiltration or extravasation of irritating or contaminated fluids or equipment.

Assessment

Signs of cellulitis are as follows:

1. Edema
2. Redness
3. Pain
4. Functional irritation

Nursing Interventions

Nursing treatment for cellulitis is similar to treatment for infiltration/extravasation.

For preventive interventions, see preventive interventions for vein irritation, phlebitis, thrombosis, thrombophlebitis, infiltration, and extravasation.

Nerve, Tendon, or Ligament Damage

Nerve, tendon, or ligament damage is related to improper techniques or extravasation of infusate. Causes include the following:

1. Penetration during intravenous insertion
2. Infiltration/extravasation of vesicants (agents causing blistering, sloughing, or necrosis) or other damaging solution
3. Cellulitis

Assessment

Assess for impaired motor or sensory function in the area of and distal to the infusion site.

Nursing Interventions

Nursing treatments following damage consist in following medical regimens as well as the orders of a physical therapist.

Preventive nursing actions include all nursing interventions for prevention of infiltration/extravasation, proper insertion and discontinuation techniques, and frequent assessment.

Hematoma

Hematoma is a mass that is produced by coagulation of extravasated blood into the tissue. Causes include the following:

1. Improper insertion technique
2. Improper discontinuation technique
3. Infiltration/extravasation

Assessment

Observe for the following:

1. Swelling at the infusion site
2. Decreased or no flow
3. Palpable firmness at site
4. Possibly redness
5. Possibly pain due to pressure of the accumulation of blood in the tissues

Nursing Interventions

Nursing treatments include the following:

1. Stop the IV immediately.
2. Apply cold packs.

Preventive interventions include the following:

1. Properly and skillfully insert the infusion device.
2. Properly discontinue the IV (see Chapter 6).
3. Prevent infiltration/extravasation.

Collapsed Vessel

A collapsed vessel takes on a flattened form since it has little, if any, blood flowing through it. Causes include the following:

1. Poor circulation
2. Too much negative pressure exerted by IV flow system or syringe

Assessment

1. Vessel wall not palpable; little or no resistance or elasticity
2. Little or no flow of IV fluid

Nursing Interventions

Nursing treatments are directed toward not using this vessel.

Preventive interventions include the following:

1. Avoid the use of vessels with poor circulation.
2. Avoid exerting negative pressure on the vessel when using a syringe.

Venous Spasm

Venous spasms are involuntary contractions of the muscles of the vessel wall. The following are three primary causes of venous spasm:

1. Infusing irritating solution
2. Infusing cold infusate
3. Vasovagal syndrome triggered by fear and apprehension

Assessment

The primary assessment parameter is decreased flow of infusate.

Nursing Interventions

Nursing treatment interventions include the following:

1. Decrease the irritating effects of the infusate by altering the flow rate to promote dilution.
2. Apply warm packs to the site if a cold infusate has been infused.
3. Provide relaxation measures.

Preventive interventions include the following:

1. Understand the degree that various solution types may be irritating (see Chapter 2).
2. If safe, allow the infusate to warm to room temperature before infusion.
3. Prevent anxiety by being a competent, skillful nurse, offering reassurance and using relaxation techniques.

Pain

The sense of suffering that is initiated by stimulation of the nerve endings describes the pain response in IV therapy patients. Two primary causes of pain are as follows:

1. Insertion of the IV needle/cannula/catheter
2. Administration of irritating medications

Assessment

Assessment consists in asking the patient to describe the discomfort. Areas to be considered are the following:

1. Where is the discomfort?
2. When did it start?
3. Is it dull, pressure, sharp, steady, intermittent?
4. What seems to make the pain diminish? Increase?

Nursing Interventions

Nursing treatment interventions are the following:

1. Decrease or increase the flow rate depending on the infusate being administered.
2. Apply warm/cold packs, depending on policy.

   Preventive interventions are as follows:

1. Teach patient proper care of the IV infusion site.
2. Employ skillful insertion techniques.
3. Properly discontinue the IV

Inaccurate Flow Rate

Inaccurate flow rates are rates that do not conform to prescribed rates of flow by being either too fast or too slow. Causes include the following:

1. IV Runouts
   - Lack of correct monitoring
   - Clamp slips
   - Patient tampers with clamp

- Change of limb position
- "Catching up"

2. Slow flow (see Chapter 4)
   - Decreased atmospheric pressure
   - Air vent obstruction
   - Bed raised too high
   - Low IV standard
   - Clot formation (fibrin sleeves)
   - "Creep" or "cold flow" of plastic tubing
   - Increased viscosity of fluid
   - Filters
   - Infiltration
   - Kinked/pinched tubing
   - Excess fills

Assessment

Assessment consists in evaluating the flow rate and factors affecting it.

Nursing Interventions

Nursing treatment interventions are as follows:

1. Determine the cause(s) of the slow or fast flow rate.
2. Correct this cause.

   Preventive interventions include the following:

1. Provide consistent and thorough patient education.
2. Secure clamps.
3. Do not "catch up" flow rate.
4. Maintain adequate height of the IV pole.
5. Use armboards.
6. See section on prevention of thrombus formation.

   Instruct the patient in the following:

1. Do not kink or compress the tubing.
2. Move the entire limb rather than only the hand/wrist.
3. Avoid using the arm/hand with the IV.
4. Do not lie on the IV arm.

5. Do not change the height of the IV pole.
6. Do not adjust the flow clamp.
7. When walking, call the nurse for assistance.
8. Call the nurse under the following circumstances:
    - You notice fluid dripping fast.
    - You notice fluid not dripping.
    - You feel wetness at the site.
    - You bump the site.

Needle/Cannula Occlusion

Blockage in the cannula or needle results in obstruction of flow. Causes include the following:

1. Fibrin sleeve formation
2. Thrombus formation at the site
3. No infusate flow (*e.g.,* empty infusate container)

A 10% fatality rate is documented if embolus results (Weinstein, 1986).

Assessment

Evaluate the flow rate for consistency to ordered rate.

Nursing Interventions

Nursing treatment interventions include the following:

1. Evaluate the cause of the occlusion.
2. Attempt to reinstate flow rate by raising the container or opening the clamp.
3. Irrigate the infusion device, if consistent with institutional policy. (See guidelines in Chapter 6.)
4. Restart the IV in another site.
5. Specific procedures have been outlined for the clearance of occlusions of central catheters using fibrinolytic therapy. Two agents most commonly used are streptokinase and urokinase. In addition, tissue plasminogen activator (TPA) is the newest agent used for clearing catheters. Guidelines for administration of

streptokinase and urokinase are the following (Weinstein, 1986):

- Streptokinase
  Put on sterile gloves.
  Initially administer 250,000 IU intravenously over 30 minutes.
  Infuse 100,000 IU/hr for 24 to 72 hours as maintenance treatment.
  Keep the patient on bed rest.
  Monitor vital signs frequently.
  Ascertain that thrombin time after 4 hours of therapy is 1½ times normal.
- Urokinase
  Put on sterile gloves.
  Gently attempt to aspirate blood from the catheter using a 10-ml syringe.
  Administer 5000 IU by way of a 1-ml tuberculin syringe at the catheter hub by injecting an amount equal to the volume of the catheter.
  Remove the syringe.
  Wait 5 minutes.
  Using a sterile 5-ml syringe, attempt to aspirate 4 ml to 5 ml of blood.
  Irrigate or flush the catheter with 0.9% normal saline.
  Remove the syringe and reconnect the IV tubing.
  If the procedure is unsuccessful, up to six attempts can be made.

Preventive interventions include the following:

1. Do not let the IV container run dry.
2. Correctly tape and position the IV needle/cannula.
3. Maintain an accurate flow rate.

Inadvertent Intra-Arterial Injection

Inadvertent intra-arterial injection occurs when fluid is injected into the artery when it was intended for injection into the vein. Causes include the following:

1. Careless technique
2. Mistaking an artery for a vein (see Table 5-1 in Chapter 5)

Assessment

1. Observe the color of the blood return (it should be dark red, not bright red).
2. Observe for direction of flow of injection (arterial flow will be away from the heart; venous flow will be toward the heart).

Nursing Interventions

Nursing treatment interventions are the following:

1. Stop the injection immediately after realizing placement is in the artery.
2. Notify the physician.

Preventive interventions include the following:

1. Know the difference between arteries and veins. Consider the following criteria:
   · Blood is bright red in an artery and dark red in a vein.
   · Arteries pulsate; veins do not.
   · Flow in arteries is away from the heart; flow in veins is toward the heart.
   · Arteries are usually located deep in muscle; veins are usually superficial.
2. Utilize meticulous care during insertion procedure.

Bibliography

Amonsen S, Gren J: Relationship between length of time and contamination in open intravenous solution. Nurs Res 27(5):372, 1978

Baciewicz A, Crass R, Robertson N: Postinfusion phlebitis associated with selected cephalosporins. Am J Intravenous Ther Clin Nutr, 9:9–14, 1982

Boyd B: The impact of a team approach on catheter-related infections. Nutritional Support Services 5(4):22, 1985

Carlson C: National phlebitis rates. NITA Update 6(6):5, 1985

Chrystal C: I.V. complication rates. NITA Update 6(3):5, 1985

Delaney C: Nurses' knowledge of selected factors that influence the IV rate. Unpublished thesis, December, 1978.

Drew D, Schumann D: Homogeneity of potassium chloride in small volume intravenous containers. Nurs Res 95(6):325, 1986

Faehnrich J: Extravasation. NITA 7(1):49, 1984

Feldstein A: Detect phlebitis and infiltration—before they harm your patient. Nursing86, 16:44–47, 1986

Germain T: A clinical evaluation of the effect of tip integrity of I.V. catheters on phlebitis rates. NITA 9(2):115, 1986

Ghildyal S, Pande R, Misra T: Histopathology and bacteriology of postinfusion phlebitis. Int Surg 60:6–7, 1975

Glister S: The impact of a team approach on catheter-related infections. Nutritional Support Services 5(4):22, 1985

Harrigan C: A cost-effective guide for the prevention of chemical phlebitis caused by the pH of the pharmaceutical agent. NITA 6(6):438, 1984

Jarmen C: Vein trauma—its complications and prevention. Intravenous Therapy News 12(7):4, 1985

Johnston-Early A, Cohen M, White K: Venipuncture and problem veins. Am J Nurs 81:1636–1640, 1981

Jones S, Koldjeski D: Clinical indicators of a developmental process in phlebitis. NITA 7:279, 1984

Larson E, Lunche S, Tran J: Correlates of I.V. phlebitis. NITA 7(3):203, 1984

Maddox R: Double-blind study to investigate methods to prevent cephalothin-induced phlebitis. Am J Hosp Pharm 34:30, 1977

Millam D: Postinfusion phlebitis. Nursing84, 14:36–37, 1984

Nurse Drug Alert: Managing extravasation wounds caused by antineoplastic drugs. NITA Update 6(6):5, 1985

Roebuck M: The effects of quality assessment on I.V. therapy. NITA 7(2):103, 1984

Roquet R, Mellies J: I.V. run-outs: Complications, costs, and prevention. NITA 6(6):438, 1983

Silverman H: Infusion phlebitis. Special Delivery 1(2):1, 1985

Trent B: The effects of utilization of an I.V. therapy team upon the incidence of I.V. peripheral-associated phlebitis. NITA 7(4):295, 1984

Tully J, Friedland G, Baldini L, Goldmann D: Complications of intravenous therapy with steel needles and Teflon® catheters. Am J Med 70:702, 1981

Turco S: Hazards associated with parenteral therapy. Am J Intravenous Ther Clin Nutr 8(10):9, 1981

Turco S: In-line filtration reduces phlebitis by two-thirds. Parenterals 3(3):2, 1985

Weinstein S: Thrombolytic therapy. NITA 9(1):31, 1986

Wetmore N: Extravasation—the dreaded complication. NITA 8(1):47, 1985

Williams D, Gibson J, Vos J, Kind A: Infusion thrombophlebitis and infiltration associated with intravenous canulae. NITA 5:379, 1982

9 ▷

Systemic Complications

Key Points

1. Septicemia, bacteremia, pyrogenic reaction
2. Circulatory overload
3. Speed shock
4. Embolism
5. Pneumothorax, hemothorax, hydrothorax
6. Hypersensitivity/allergic reactions

Common systemic complications of IV therapy include the following:

Septicemia, Bacteremia, Pyrogenic Reaction

1. *Septicemia* is defined as systemic infection in the circulating blood resulting from pathogens spread from an infection in some part of the body.
2. *Bacteremia* is defined as the presence of bacteria in the bloodstream.
3. *Pyrogenic reaction* is a term given to the fever response caused by some substance or agent. These substances can be metabolic products of living organisms or the dead microorganisms themselves. If this reaction occurs in response to an infusate or type of equipment, the response will usually be evident within 30 minutes of infusion of such substance.
4. Some of the most common infecting organisms are *Klebsiella pneumoniae, Enterobacter cloacae, Staphylococcus aureus,* and the fungal organism of *Candida albicans.*

5. Causes of septicemia include the following:
   - Prolonged IV therapy
   - Breaks in aseptic technique
   - Flaws in equipment
   - Contaminated equipment
   - Contaminated infusate
6. Indwelling catheters can be a significant source of infection.

Assessment

Assess for the following signs and symptoms:

1. Chills
2. Fever
3. Headache
4. Backache
5. Prostration
6. Nausea
7. Vomiting
8. Diarrhea
9. Cyanosis
10. Syncope
11. Shortness of breath
12. Shock signs/symptoms

The signs and symptoms for pyrogenic reaction usually appear within 30 minutes after the infusion is started.

Nursing Interventions

Treatment interventions are the following:

1. Slow the infusion.
2. Immediately stop the infusion if the fever response is immediate.
3. Notify the physician.
4. Continuously monitor vital signs.
5. Save the infusate and all equipment so it can be tested for pathogens.
6. Look for all possible sources of contamination.

Preventive interventions to prevent septicemia and pyrogenic reaction are the following:

1. Maintain meticulous aseptic techniques.
2. Keep all IV sites clean, dry, and covered.
3. Continuously and thoroughly assess patient status.
4. Routinely monitor the temperature in all IV therapy patients.
5. Thoroughly evaluate all equipment and solutions used.
6. Note all the interventions for prevention of vein irritation and phlebitis.

Circulatory Overload

Circulatory overload is an excess in the extracellular fluid volume. Causes include the following:

1. Infusing an excessive amount of saline solution
2. Infusing saline infusate too fast
3. Infusing saline infusate at night when the functioning of the renal system is diminished

Assessment

Signs and symptoms of circulatory overload include the following:

1. Weight gain
2. Pitting edema
3. Puffy eyelids
4. Flushed face
5. Shock
6. Hypertension
7. Increased respiration
8. Ascites
9. Distention of neck veins
10. Increased venous pressure
11. Gradual increase in pulse
12. Cyanosis

In addition, observe for the signs and symptoms of pulmonary edema, which include rapid, shallow breathing; restlessness; apprehension; pale color; cyanosis; pink, frothy sputum; increased pulse; increased blood pressure; and possibly edema of extremities.

Nursing Interventions

Nursing treatment interventions are as follows:

1. Slow the infusion to a KVO (keep open) rate.
2. Notify the physician.
3. Continuously and carefully monitor the vital signs every 30 minutes.
4. Elevate the patient's head.
5. Monitor the flow rate.
6. Be prepared to respond to the symptoms of pulmonary edema.

Preventive interventions are as follows:

1. Weigh IV patients daily.
2. Strictly monitor IV flow rate.
3. Use controllers and pumps as appropriate.
4. Do not "catch up" IVs that are behind schedule.
5. Do not overload the kidneys at night by infusing large amounts of fluid. Because blood pressure decreases during sleep, kidney filtration decreases.
6. Monitor output.

Speed Shock

Speed shock is a sudden severe systemic reaction to IV medications that were administered too rapidly by either bolus or infusion, or in excessive amounts.

Assessment

Speed shock includes the following signs and symptoms:

1. Flushed face
2. Pounding headache

3. Hypertension
4. Sudden increase in pulse
5. Irregular pulse
6. Possible loss of consciousness
7. Apprehension
8. Chills
9. Dyspnea
10. Possible cardiac arrest
11. The signs and symptoms of the drug administered

Nursing Interventions

Immediate treatment interventions are as follows:
1. Slow or stop the infusion.
2. Check vital signs.
3. Evaluate circulatory and neurologic status.
4. Notify the physician.

   Preventive interventions are as follows:

1. Carefully monitor the flow rate and the patient's responses to infusate and medications.
2. Know the actions and side effects of the drug being administered.
3. Use IV pumps when indicated.
4. Maintain the infusion rate as prescribed.

Embolism

Embolism is an abnormal circulatory condition in which a blood clot or foreign body travels and becomes lodged in a blood vessel. Types include air, catheter, clot, and hair emboli.

1. Air embolism results from entry of air into the venous infusion line as a result of the IV running dry, air in the tubing, air in syringes used for drug administration, and negative pressure at sites located in the head, neck, and shoulders.
2. Catheter embolism results from a portion of the catheter breaking away, and moving in the venous system.

3. Clot embolism results from a blood clot developing, breaking away from the vessel wall or catheter, and moving in the venous system. This can also result from irrigation of the infusion device. Review Chapter 8 for the causes of thrombus formation.
4. Hair embolism results from a hair being severed by the infusion device on insertion.

Assessment

The signs and symptoms of embolism are dependent on where the embolism lodges and the degree of occlusion resulting. General signs and symptoms follow:

1. Cyanosis
2. Hypotension
3. Increased pulse
4. Increased venous pressure
5. Fainting and possible loss of consciousness

Nursing Interventions

Treatment interventions are the following:

1. Place a tourniquet above the site (proximal to the venipuncture site) if catheter embolism is suspected.
2. Turn the patient on the left side with the head lower than the heart and place in Trendelenburg's position if air embolism is suspected.
3. Stress complete bed rest.
4. Monitor vital signs.
5. Administer oxygen for air embolism.
6. Notify the physician.

Preventive interventions for air embolism:

1. Secure all connections to prevent air from entering the infusion system.
2. Use the Valsalva maneuver when changing tubing on central lines.
3. Use clamps during tubing changes.
4. Use air-eliminating filters.

5. Fill the drip chamber before filling tubing.
6. Prime tubing "up" rather than "down," where applicable. (See Chapter 5 for explanation of technique.)
7. Remove all air from syringes, tubing.
8. Maintain flow rate to prevent a dry IV.
9. Use Luer Locks and other securing devices where applicable.

Preventive interventions for catheter embolism:

1. Check catheters/cannulas for defects prior to insertion.
2. Use radiopaque catheters.
3. Do not remove and then reinsert stylet during insertion.
4. Anchor the infusion device securely.
5. Note the length of the catheter on insertion and removal, and document this information.

Preventive interventions for thrombus:

1. Avoid irrigating the administration system. (See Chapter 8 for guidelines for prevention of vein irritation.)

Preventive interventions for hair embolism:

1. Remove hair from the insertion site by clipping or using a depilatory prior to initiating therapy.

Pneumothorax, Hemothorax, Hydrothorax

Complications such as pneumothorax, hemothorax, and hydrothorax are related to the use of central lines. Refer to Chapter 12 for description.

Hypersensitivity/Allergic Reactions

Hypersensitivity reaction is an inappropriate and excessive response of the immune system to a sensitizing antigen. Such a response in IV therapy can be attributed to sensitivity to the infusate or medications added.

Causes include sensitivity to the following:

1. Infusate (*e.g.,* glucose solution, fat emulsions containing egg products)
2. Medication
3. Preservatives, including reactions to the following:
   - Sodium bisulfate in dialysis solution
   - Phenol in glucagon
   - Sodium benzoate in diazepam
   - Benzyl alcohol from saline solution

Assessment

Signs and symptoms may include but are not limited to the following:

1. Urticaria
2. Eczema
3. Dyspnea
4. Bronchospasm
5. Diarrhea
6. Rhinitis
7. Sinusitis
8. Anaphylaxis

Nursing Interventions

Treatment interventions are as follows:

1. Discontinue the infusion.
2. Carefully monitor the vital signs.
3. Notify the physician.

The primary preventive intervention is to thoroughly assess the patient's history for any factors related to allergies and communicate such information to those involved in administering therapy. In addition, thorough observation of the patient when any infusate or medication is administered for the first time is necessary. However, note that any patient may experience an idiosyncratic reaction (*i.e.,* a reaction completely unique to that person at that time). For example, the patient may never have experienced hypersensitivity to a particular medication on previous administrations but does at this particular time.

Bibliography

Estner M, Goldfarb I, Savini M et al: Internal jugular vein thrombosis. NITA 9(3):220, 1986

Feldstein A: Catheter embolus. Nursing85 15:59, 1985

Metheny N: The interstitial (third-space) phenomenon. NITA 6(4):251, 1983

Warren J: Edema—a serious I.V. complication. NITA 7(4):277, 1984

Weinstein S: Thrombolytic therapy. NITA 9(1):31, 1986

Unit IV

Parenteral Nutrition

10 ▷ Nutritional Assessment

Key Points

1. Basics of nutrition
2. Assessment of nutritional status:
   - Patient history
   - Physical assessment overview
   - Anthropomorphic measurements
   - Laboratory tests useful for assessment of nutrition
3. Patients at risk for protein–calorie malnutrition

Basics of Nutrition

The basic principles of nutrition note that both energy and protein, as well as water and a variety of fats, minerals, and vitamins, are essential to maintain adequate nutrition. The most common occurrences of inadequate nutrition, or malnutrition, are protein and energy deficits, commonly called protein–calorie malnutrition. Protein-calorie malnutrition has been documented to exist in 30% to 50% of hospitalized patients (Butterworth and Weinsier, 1980). These statistics support the need for healthcare providers to be knowledgeable about nutritional needs and adept at nutritional assessment. Assessment of nutritional status forms the foundation of initiating and monitoring parenteral nutrition.

Energy and Protein

Both energy and protein are required for adequate nutrition. If energy (calories) and protein supply to the body are inadequate, the body uses its first backup energy supply, the glycogen reserve, to overcome the deficit. This glycogen reserve may last for approximately 1 day before it is depleted. The body then attempts to use free fatty acids mobilized from adipose tissue as an energy source. Utilization of this second energy source can be slowed by an increase in insulin secretion in response to various types of stress, such as sepsis, injury, or hypermetabolism. If insulin levels rise high enough, ketone production by the liver will be suppressed and the body will then turn to a third energy source: protein.

The two protein pools from which energy can be derived are the following:

1. *Visceral protein pool*. Includes serum circulating protein substances of albumin and transferrin
2. *Somatic protein pool*. Includes the protein in skeletal and smooth muscle as well as in structural tissues

The visceral protein pool is used by the body before the somatic protein pool. That is, the patient's serum albumin and transferrin concentrations will decrease before there is any significant drop in body weight, which would demonstrate muscle loss from the somatic protein pool.

Protein–Calorie Malnutrition

Protein–calorie malnutrition can exist in the following two states:

1. *Marasmus*. This type of malnutrition is characterized by decreased intake of calories with adequate amounts of protein intake. Although the visceral protein pool remains intact, a decrease in body fat or muscle mass from the somatic protein pool occurs.
2. *Kwashiorkor*. This type of malnutrition is characterized by an adequate calorie intake with inadequate

amounts of protein intake. Although the somatic protein pool remains intact, the visceral protein pool is depleted.

Assessment of Nutritional Status

Assessment of nutritional status is essential for correcting or preventing malnutrition. Based on the foregoing discussion, several areas of assessment are used to determine nutritional status.

Patient History

1. A thorough assessment of current as well as normal body height and weight is necessary to determine any significant weight loss.
2. Patterns of oral intake, including the ability to secure and prepare food and ingest and digest food, provide insight into the total picture of nutritional need.
3. Psychosocial dimensions of nutrition, including personal, ethnic, and religious food preferences, financial concerns, emotional responses related to pain, motivation, and perception, should be assessed.

Physical Assessment Overview

A general review of all body systems is essential in completing a thorough nutritional assessment. Observation of the hair, nails, skin, mucous membranes, teeth, and mouth are especially significant.

Anthropomorphic Measurements

Anthropomorphic measurements are made to determine changes in protein and energy stores in the body that are reflected in fat stores and muscle mass.

1. Determining body weight is an essential anthropomorphic measurement indicative of changes in the somatic protein pool and body fat. The percentage of ideal body weight that the actual body weight reflects is a frequent measurement. This percentage is deter-

mined by subtracting the patient's actual body weight from the ideal body weight determined from a standardized chart. This amount is then divided by the ideal body weight, and the result is multiplied by 100. If this percentage is greater than 90%, the state of nutrition is considered normal. As the percentage decreases, the degree of malnutrition progresses from mild at 80% to 90%, down to severe malnutrition at 60% to 70%. It should be noted that the best approach for using weight measures is to identify the actual body weight and monitor changes over time.

2. A second anthropomorphic measurement is the triceps skinfold thickness (TST). This measures stored body fat. A caliper is used to measure the skinfold covering the mid-upper arm. Since the compressibility of fat differs from person to person, the measurement can be affected.

3. Mid-arm circumference (MAC) reflects the patient's lean body mass or skeletal muscle mass. Use the same midpoint in the arm as that selected for the TST and measure the circumference of the arm.

4. The mid-arm muscle circumference (MAMC) reflects both fat deposits and skeletal muscle or lean body mass and is calculated by using both the MAC and the TST measurements according to the following formula:

$$MAMC = MAC - (0.314 \times TST)$$

Laboratory Tests Useful for Assessment of Nutrition

1. The creatinine/height index (CHI) is a measure of somatic protein stores. The amount of creatinine in the body is directly proportional to the amount of muscle present in the body. The CHI is calculated according to this formula:

$$CHI = \frac{\text{actual urinary creatinine}}{\text{expected urinary creatinine}} \times 100$$

This value is then compared with normal standards that are based on the patient's height to determine the degree of deficiency. Patients with malnutrition will have abnormally low levels, reflecting loss of lean body mass.

2. The visceral protein stores are evaluated by measuring the serum albumin and serum transferrin levels. In the malnourished patient these levels decrease. The normal serum albumin value is 4 g to 4.5 g/dl. Normal levels of serum transferrin are approximately 180 mg to 200 mg/dl. Albumin levels less than 2.5 g to 3 g/dl and transferrin levels less than 140 mg to 160 mg/dl may signify moderate malnutrition.

3. Laboratory tests that measure immune system function are sometimes used to evaluate nutritional status. Total lymphocyte count (TLC) is depressed in patients with malnutrition. A value below $1500/mm^3$ can be indicative of malnourishment.

4. Skin testing is also employed to evaluate the immune system. Antigens frequently used to measure reactivity include mumps antigen, trichophytin, candidin, purified protein derivative (PPD), coccidioidin, and histoplasmin. In the malnourished patient the skin response is usually delayed or absent. It is important to remember that a number of variables can affect the cellular immune response (drugs, stress, sensitivity), all potentially causing a false reading. Skin testing is at best a *general* test to indicate nutritional status.

In summary, a variety of tools and methods are available to evaluate nutritional status and diagnose protein–calorie malnutrition. Newer methods for assessment of nutritional status include carbon dioxide consumption, neuron activation, and sodium–potassium balance. Regardless of the methods chosen, it is essential to select a variety of tests and measurements rather than relying on any one test.

Patients at Risk for Protein–Calorie Malnutrition

1. Grossly underweight patients (weight for height below 80% of standard)

2. Grossly overweight patients (weight for height above 120% of standard)—an often overlooked malnutrition in acutely ill patients
3. Patients with recent weight loss greater than 10% of usual body weight
4. Alcoholics
5. Patients with no oral intake for more than 10 days, including those receiving standard 5% dextrose IV fluids for this period
6. Preoperative/postoperative patients, especially those with gastrointestinal disturbances
7. Patients with protracted nutrient losses such as malabsorption syndromes, short gut syndromes/fistulas, renal dialysis, draining wounds, abscesses
8. Patients with increased metabolic needs such as those with extensive burns, sepsis, protracted fever, or trauma
9. Patients receiving drugs with antinutrient or catabolic properties, such as steroids, immunosuppressants, or antitumor drugs

Bibliography

Bloch AS: Developing nutrition screening/assessment forms. Am J Intravenous Ther Clin Nutr 7:17–25, 1980

Butterworth CE, Weinsier RL: Malnutrition in hospitalized patients: Assessment and treatment. In Goodhart RS, Shils ME (eds): Modern Nutrition in Health and Disease, 6th ed. Philadelphia, Lea & Febiger, 1980

Kaminski MV, JeeJeebhoy KN: Nutritional assessment—diagnosis of malnutrition and selection of therapy. Am J Intravenous Ther Clin Nutr 7:12–23, 1980

Koelting CA, Schneider PJ: Pros and cons of anthropomorphic measurements. Infusion 9(6):184, 1985

Schneider PJ: Factors supporting the use of total parenteral nutrition. Am J Intravenous Ther Clin Nutr 7:35–45, 1980

Schneider PJ: Skin tests and nutrition. Infusion 7:151, 1983

11 ▷ Administration of Parenteral Nutrition

Key Points

1. Routes for delivery and indications for use
2. Catheters available
3. Infusate considerations
4. Patient education
5. Administration techniques

Routes for Delivery and Indications for Use

Once it has been established that a patient is malnourished and in need of nutritional support (see Chapter 10 for nutritional assessment techniques), the physician will decide which form the nutritional support will take. Usually enteral nutrition (diets in fluid form administered through a tube into the gastrointestinal tract) is the preferred method owing to its lower cost and lower rate of complications (Pestana, 1985). However, for the many patients who cannot tolerate tube feedings or who are not consuming food orally for certain reasons, parenteral nutrition (PN) can be selected as an alternative mode of therapy.

Reasons for Parenteral Nutrition

The following situations may warrant the use of parenteral nutrition (Griggs, 1984):

1. Altered metabolic states often found in hepatic insufficiency or renal failure

2. Inadequate gastrointestinal function as seen in short-bowel syndrome, ileus, malabsorption, or pancreatitis
3. Trauma- or sepsis-induced hypermetabolic states

Approaches

There are two basic approaches to the administration of parenteral nutrition.

1. Peripheral venous nutrition (PVN)
   - Can be given through a standard peripheral catheter
   - Used for patients having simple or short-term supplemental nutritional requirements lasting less than 1 week
   - Can be used when a central venous catheter is contraindicated owing to coagulopathy, venous thrombosis, or sepsis
   - Site usually rotated every 48 to 72 hours
   - Can be supplemental to oral intake
   - Can be supplemental to enteral feeding
2. Central venous nutrition (CVN)
   - Can be given through a peripherally inserted catheter positioned in a central vein, or through a surgically placed central venous catheter
   - Used for long-term therapy and in home-care setting
   - Various catheter types and insertion sites available
   - Useful in treatment of a variety of disease entities:
     Malnourished patients prior to major surgery
     Gastrointestinal syndromes: fistula, malabsorption, pancreatitis, inflammatory bowel disease, short-bowel syndrome
     Renal or hepatic failure
     Neoplastic disease with gastrointestinal toxicity due to chemotherapy

Catheters Available

A variety of vascular access devices are available for the delivery of parenteral nutrition as well as other solutions.

Standard Peripheral IV Catheters

(See Chapter 3 for a description of these devices.)

Small-Gauge Peripheral Central Venous Catheters

An example is the Intrasil catheter by Travenol Laboratories.

Features
1. Can be peripherally placed but central venous access is achieved
2. Average size 15 gauge and 50 cm to 60 cm in length
3. Silicone elastomer material is biocompatible and infrequently associated with fibrin sheath formation or phlebitis (Bottino et al, 1979)
4. Tip of catheter rests in the superior vena cava; catheter can be sutured in place
5. Radiopaque

Uses
1. Alternative to subclavian venipuncture
2. Provides venous access for single, intermittent, or continuous infusions
3. Advantageous for short-term therapy

Advantages
1. Can be inserted as a nonsurgical procedure
2. Can remain in place longer than a standard peripheral catheter
3. Spares the patient repeated vein sticks for intermittent injections and infusions
4. Is easily removed by gentle pulling with steady tension

Disadvantages
1. Requires daily maintenance, including site care and heparin flushing if the device will be intermittent
2. Not usually accessible for blood drawing because of small diameter of catheter

Small-Gauge Central Venous Catheters

Examples are the Centrasil catheter by Travenol Laboratories and the Arrow Multi-Lumen Catheter System by Arrow International, Inc.

Features
1. Centrally placed, usually in the subclavian vein
2. Size varies from 15 to 18 gauge and 15 cm to 30 cm in length
3. Silicone elastomer or polyurethane material is biocompatible and infrequently associated with fibrin sheath formation or phlebitis (Bottino, 1979; Linder, 1984)
4. Tip of catheter rests in the superior vena cava; catheter can be sutured in place
5. Radiopaque
6. Multilumen catheters can dedicate different lumina to different solutions/purposes

Uses
1. Provides venous access for single, intermittent, or continuous infusions, by subclavian venipuncture
2. Used for short-term or long-term therapy
3. Blood drawing usually discouraged with small-diameter single-lumen catheters, but multilumen catheters can dedicate a lumen for this purpose

Advantages
1. Can usually be inserted as a nonsurgical procedure
2. Can remain in place for long periods
3. Spares the patient repeated vein sticks for intermittent injections and infusions

4. Is easily removed by gentle pulling with steady tension

Disadvantages
1. Complications associated with direct subclavian venipuncture (see Chapter 12)
2. Daily maintenance necessary, including site care and heparin flushing if the device will be intermittent

Silicone Silastic Long-Term Indwelling Atrial Catheters: Hickman and Broviac by Evermed

Features
1. The Hickman catheter is made of silicone rubber, is white, is opaque, and measures 90 cm in length; it has an internal diameter of 1.6 mm (the larger diameter makes blood drawing possible) and is available with one or two Dacron cuffs.
2. The Broviac catheter differs from the Hickman in that it has a smaller internal diameter of 1 mm. It is made of silicone rubber and is 90 cm in length. Modified versions are available for neonates and pediatric patients.
3. A recent modification is the double-lumen Hickman catheter in which a Hickman and a Broviac are fused together.
4. These catheters are placed into a large vein (cephalic, internal or external jugular) with the tip of the catheter resting in the right atrium.
5. A Dacron cuff situated 30 cm from the hub of the catheter serves to seal the subcutaneous tunnel used during catheter placement and to promote fibrosis that helps secure the catheter in place.
6. The external end of the catheter has a Luer lock hub that allows for the addition of several types of available adapters.
7. Insertion can usually be done on an inpatient or outpatient basis using local or general anesthesia.
8. Removal of the catheter is generally uncomplicated using steady tension, but occasionally blunt dissec-

tion of the cuff from the subcutaneous tissues is necessary.

Uses
1. Intended for long-term venous access with intermittent or continuous IV administration
2. A variety of solutions can be infused through these catheters: replacement fluids, parenteral nutrition, chemotherapy, antibiotics, and blood products; in addition, the catheters may be used for plasmapheresis and for blood drawing.

Advantages
1. Versatility
2. Ease of use without patient discomfort

Disadvantages
1. Most serious potential problem is infection
2. Daily maintenance necessary, including site care and heparin flushing if the device will be intermittent
3. Catheter exit site in the anterior chest disagreeable cosmetically to some patients

Silicone Silastic Long-Term Indwelling Atrial Catheter: Groshong by Catheter Technology Corporation

Features
1. First introduced in 1985, this thin-walled catheter is made of translucent silicone rubber; the tip of the catheter is rounded and closed, with an adjacent two-way slit valve that opens outwardly to allow infusion; when the infusion is completed, the valve closes, eliminating the need for clamping.
2. Withdrawal of blood is possible through the catheter since the slit valve opens inwardly with negative pressure; this also allows for central venous pressure monitoring without retrograde blood flow.
3. The catheter is placed in the vessel and then subcuta-

neously tunneled to an exit site, much like the Hickman catheter.
4. The connector on the external end of the catheter is a push fit design.

Uses
1. Same as for the Hickman and Broviac catheters

Advantages
1. Clamping not required
2. Heparin flushes not required to remain patency (a 5-ml saline flush after each administration or once a week maintains patency; a 20-ml saline flush is recommended after blood infusion or withdrawal)
3. Not subject to air embolism or accidental blood loss

Disadvantages
1. Most serious potential problem is infection
2. Daily maintenance of site necessary
3. Catheter exit site in the anterior chest disagreeable cosmetically to some patients

Totally Implantable Venous Access Ports

Currently three devices are available: the Mediport (by Cormed), the Infuse-A-Port (by Infusaid), and the Port-a-Cath (by Pharmacia).

Features
1. The system consists of a self-sealing silicone rubber injection port connected to a Silastic catheter.
2. The port is usually placed in a subcutaneous pocket made over a bony prominence, and the catheter is tunneled to a central vein leading into the right atrium.
3. The insertion position is confirmed by fluoroscopy; the port is flushed with heparinized saline and sutured to the underlying fascia before the incisions are closed.

4. The port is easily palpable and may be used immediately after insertion.
5. A specially designed Huber needle that reduces coring of the silicone rubber septum is used to enter the device through the skin; a right-angle needle is used for continuous infusion and a straight needle for bolus infusion.

Uses
These ports are highly versatile and can be used to:

1. Deliver chemotherapeutic drugs, parenteral nutrition, antibiotics, and blood and blood products
2. Draw blood samples

Advantages
1. Implantable ports require no daily maintenance between use; they are flushed vigorously with heparinized saline every 28 days to maintain patency (Goodman and Wickham, 1984).
2. Because these devices are totally subcutaneous, they require no dressings; patients can swim or bathe without taking any special precautions and find the device to be aesthetically acceptable.

Disadvantages
1. Reported complications include catheter rupture, dislodgement of the catheter from the septum, infection, occlusion, and extravasation from improper needle placement (Foltz, 1987; Lokich *et al,* 1985).
2. Blood drawing may be problematic with the smaller ports.
3. Some patients experience pain on needle insertion.
4. Patients can accidentally displace the catheter by "twiddling" their portals (Gebarski and Geþarski, 1984).

Infusate Considerations

In planning to meet a patient's nutritional requirements with parenteral nutrition, several components and issues must be considered when the physician formulates therapy.

Carbohydrates

1. The most common carbohydrate used is dextrose.
2. The dextrose concentration in parenteral nutrition fluids can range from as little as 5% in peripherally administered fluids to as much as 45% in fluids administered through a central line for patients with high caloric needs or volume restriction requirements.

Protein

1. The calorie/nitrogen ratio requirement in an unstressed patient ranges from 100 to 150 nonprotein calories per gram of nitrogen; in a severely stressed or traumatized patient the required ratio could be 85 : 1 owing to glucose intolerance; renal failure patients who may not be able to tolerate protein might require a ratio of 400 : 1.
2. Protein is usually provided in parenteral nutrition at the basal rate of 0.8 g/kg/day.
3. Increased need for protein by the body is usually reflected in an increase in the excretion of urinary nitrogen.
4. Crystalline amino acid concentrations most frequently used to provide protein requirements are 4.25% and 5%, with higher concentrations being used in cases of fluid restriction or increased protein need.
5. Special amino acid formulations have been developed for use in certain disease states:
    - Essential amino acids for patients with renal failure
    - Branched chain amino acids for patients with hepatic encephalopathy
    - Certain branched chain amino acid formulations for patients who are highly stressed by injury or sepsis

Fat

1. There are several important benefits to be gained from the administration of fat.
    - When fat provides at least 4% of total caloric intake, certain complications associated with essential fatty acid deficiency (EFAD) can be prevented:
      Impaired wound healing
      Platelet dysfunction
      Increased susceptibility to infection
      Development of fatty liver
    - In patients with respiratory failure, administration of fat can help decrease carbon dioxide excretion.
    - Use of fat can help control hyperglycemia.
2. Up to 60% of total caloric intake can be given in the form of fat.
3. Fat emulsion is available in 10% and 20% concentrations and provides 1.1 calories/ml and 2 calories/ml, respectively.
4. Since fat emulsions are iso-osmolar, they can be given through either peripheral or central veins.
5. Considerations for the administration of fat emulsion are the following:
    - Peripheral administration is thought to decrease the number of entries into the central venous catheter.
    - Fat must not be infused through a micropore filter because fat particles are large (approximately 0.5 μ) and will clog most 0.22-μ IV filters; give fat emulsions through a separate IV or piggyback through a Y connector close to the phlebotomy site.
    - Before administration, give a test dose of 1 ml/min to check for adverse reaction to fat emulsion product.
    - Fat administration may be contraindicated in the following:
      Patients with pancreatitis

     Patients with fat metabolism abnormalities
     Infants with hyperbilirubinemia

3-in-1 Admixture Approach

Dextrose, amino acids, and fat are combined in one container and administered through one delivery system.

Advantages
1. Number of catheter entries decreased
2. Potential for touch contamination decreased
3. More optimal physiologic feeding provided
4. Conservation of nursing time
5. Potentially cost-effective

Disadvantages
1. Inability to use a final filter for the solution containing fat
2. Potential fat emulsion stability problems
3. Fluid and electrolyte changes must usually be made peripherally

Electrolytes

1. Most amino acid solutions differ in their electrolyte content.
2. As the patient's condition changes electrolyte requirements will vary.
   - Potassium and phosphorus needs increase during administration of a high dextrose load.
   - Magnesium and calcium needs increase when an anabolic state is established.
   - Acetate or lactate salts may be substituted for chloride salts to prevent hyperchloremic acidosis.
3. Suggested daily requirement ranges for selected electrolytes are listed below.
   - Potassium, 30 mEq to 200 mEq
   - Sodium, 50 mEq to 250 mEq
   - Magnesium, 10 mEq to 30 mEq
   - Chloride, 50 mEq to 250 mEq

- Phosphorus, 10 mmol to 40 mmol
- Calcium, 10 mEq to 20 mEq

Vitamins

1. The Nutritional Advisory Group of the American Medical Association (AMA) has developed recommendations for the daily administration of IV multivitamins (AMA, 1979):
   - A, 3300 IU
   - D, 200 IU
   - E, 10 IU
   - Ascorbic acid (C), 100 mg
   - Folic acid, 400 μg
   - Niacin (B_5), 40 mg
   - Riboflavin (B_2), 3.6 mg
   - Thiamin (B_1), 3 mg
   - Pyridoxine (B_6), 4 mg
   - Cyanocobalamin (B_{12}), 5 μg
   - Pantothenic acid (B_3), 15 mg
   - Biotin (B_7), 60 μg
2. In addition, vitamin K, 5 mg/wk, is usually given intramuscularly.
3. Stress or trauma increases a patient's need for vitamins.
4. Lipid-soluble vitamins may accumulate if excessive amounts are given.

Trace Elements

1. The AMA has also established guidelines for the daily administration of four trace elements (AMA, 1979):
   - Zinc, 2.5 mg to 4.0 mg
   - Copper, 0.5 mg to 1.5 mg
   - Chromium, 10 μg to 15 μg
   - Manganese, 0.15 mg to 0.8 mg
2. These recommended daily amounts may not ensure an adequate intake, so patient's levels should be monitored and levels adjusted accordingly.

(Continued)

3. Other trace elements that may be of benefit but for which no guidelines for administration have been established include the following:
   - Selenium
   - Iodine
   - Molybdenum
   - Fluorine
   - Cobalt
   - Nickel
   - Iron

Drugs

1. Some patients may benefit from the addition of insulin to the solution to control blood glucose levels; close patient monitoring is recommended (Woolfson et al, 1979).
2. Heparin and cortisol have been added to the solutions in an attempt to prevent fibrin sheath formation on the catheter and to reduce phlebitis (Hardin, 1983).
3. Other drugs such as certain antibiotics, cimetidine, and certain cardiac medications have been shown to be compatible with parenteral nutrition solutions, but careful consideration should be made before adding any of these drugs to the solution (Hardin, 1983).

Solution Preparation

1. All parenteral nutrition solutions should be prepared by trained personnel under a laminar flow hood using strict aseptic technique.
2. Solutions should be refrigerated until shortly before use.

Patient Education

Patients who will be receiving parenteral nutrition will understandably feel anxious about many aspects of the situation. One of the primary responsibilities of the nurse is to reduce this anxiety through careful and thorough patient teaching.

Patient education topics to be covered in preparing hospital patients (see Chapter 16 for topics related to outpatient and home parenteral therapy) to receive parenteral nutrition include the following:

1. Definition of parenteral nutrition
2. Reasons for treatment with parenteral nutrition
3. Effect of parenteral nutrition on previous nutritional habits
4. What to expect during and after the catheter insertion procedure
   - Explanation of all procedures that will be performed, approximate length of time the procedures will take, and what sensations the patient can expect to feel

     Possible need for light sedation of patient prior to catheter insertion

     Explanation of aseptic technique: gloves, gowns, masks (for patient also), preparation of insertion site, sterile drapes, and so forth

     Administration of anesthetic—expectation of pain from lidocaine (Xylocaine) injection

     The search for the subclavian vein often produces a feeling of pressure and sometimes pain.
   - Explanation of and actual practice of Valsalva maneuver and Trendelenburg position (if these will be needed during insertion)
   - Expectation of postinsertion radiograph
   - Familiarization with how the catheter will look after insertion and how it may alter body image and activity level
   - Expectation of daily regimen for care of the insertion site, tubing change protocols, and monitoring schedules
   - Patients may want to know how the catheter will be removed following their course of therapy.
5. The patient should be encouraged at all times to ask questions concerning any aspect of parenteral nutri-

tion; when feedback is elicited the nurse is able to assess the patient's level of understanding.

6. The patient's knowledge and practice of expected procedures help curb anxiety and promote a feeling of helping rather than of helplessness.

Administration Techniques

Aseptic Technique

1. All catheter care must incorporate strict aseptic technique to reduce the possibility of infectious complications.
2. The commitment of the entire institution to the highest standard of care must be encouraged.
3. Protocols specifying aseptic technique for handling the catheter, entry site, administration sets, and solutions should be written and enforced.
4. Patients receiving parenteral nutrition are at increased risk for septic complications because of the following:
   - Nutritionally deficient patients are immunologically compromised.
   - The skin as a barrier against infection is no longer intact.
   - Parenteral solutions are excellent growth media for microorganisms.
5. Special attention should be given to the encouragement and enforcement of proper handwashing technique prior to any IV therapy procedure.
6. Model standards are available from the Centers for Disease Control and from the National Intravenous Therapy Association (Colley et al, 1981; NITA, 1982; Simmons, 1982).

Insertion of Peripheral Catheters

(See Chapter 5 for peripheral catheter insertion techniques.)

Insertion of Central Venous Catheters

Subclavian venipuncture is usually performed at the patient's bedside under local anesthesia by percutaneous techniques.

Nursing Interventions

1. Attention to aseptic technique—the nurse should take the initiative in maintaining asepsis during the procedure.
2. Provide the proper equipment.
   - Proper IV administration set
   - Proper IV solution
   - Assemble set and prime tubing
3. Position the patient correctly.
   - Place the patient in Trendelenburg's position.
   - Elevate the clavicle with a towel roll placed along the thoracic vertebrae.
   - At the proper time ask the patient to perform the Valsalva maneuver.
4. Provide comfort and support to the patient by maintaining eye contact and holding the patient's hand.
5. After catheter insertion, begin to infuse isotonic IV solution and apply a sterile dressing to the site.
6. Observe the patient for signs of early complications by taking vital signs frequently, paying particular attention to respiratory rate and bilateral breath sounds. (See Chapter 12 for a discussion of complications.)
7. Arrange for a radiograph to be taken to check for proper catheter tip placement in the superior vena cava, and identify any early complications such as pneumothorax or hemothorax.

Insertion of Hickman, Broviac, and Groshong Catheters and Implantable Venous Access Ports

1. Insertion is usually done in the operating room or special procedures unit with the patient receiving local or general anesthesia.

2. Follow institutional protocol for the nurse's role in placement of these venous access devices.

Site Care and Dressing Changes

Peripheral Catheters

(See Chapters 5 and 6 for peripheral catheter site care and dressing change techniques.)

Central Venous Catheters

1. Subclavian catheter sites should be observed and gauze dressings changed at least every 48 to 72 hours or as necessary. For patients with transparent dressings, the site should be inspected through the dressing at least every 48 to 72 hours, and the transparent dressing should be changed every 4 to 7 days (Schwartz-Fulton et al, 1981; Maki and Will, 1984).

2. During site care and dressing change procedures, some institutions suggest that the nurse wear a clean gown, mask, and sterile gloves and suggest that the patient also wear a mask.

3. Sterile dressings can include traditional paper–adhesive tape dressings or semipermeable, waterproof transparent dressings.

4. Several studies have been done comparing the various dressing types with the incidence of phlebitis. Some have suggested an increased risk or incidence of problems associated with transparent dressing use (Ganz et al, 1984; Powell et al, 1982). Others have found no increased risk of phlebitis or infection when transparent dressings were worn up to 7 days (Lawson et al, 1986; Maki and Will, 1984; Schwartz-Fulton et al, 1981).

5. An example of a procedure for site care and dressing change follows:
   - Follow strict aseptic technique.
   - Wash hands with antiseptic soap.
   - Assemble necessary equipment (Fig. 11-1).
   - Using sterile gloves, remove old dressing and inspect site for any signs of infection (Fig. 11-2). Erythema

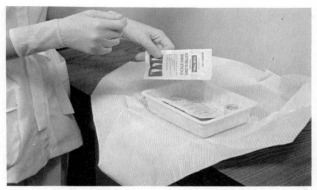

Figure 11-1. Assemble necessary equipment.

Swelling
Serous, serosanguineous, or purulent drainage
- Dispose of contaminated gloves and supplies. Wash hands and put on sterile gloves.
- Defat area with acetone alcohol and then cleanse area with antiseptic solution, always moving from the point of catheter insertion to the outside using a circular motion (Fig. 11-3).

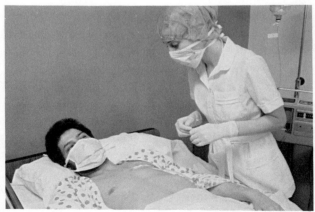

Figure 11-2. Remove old dressing.

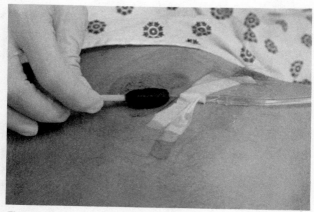

Figure 11-3. Cleanse the area.

- Allow to dry.
- Antiseptic ointment can be applied to the insertion site.
- Apply a new sterile dressing and secure in place (Fig. 11-4).
- Chart (Fig. 11-5).

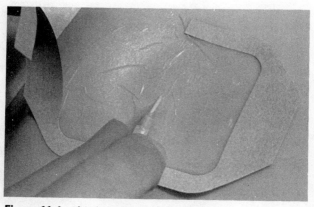

Figure 11-4. Apply a new sterile dressing.

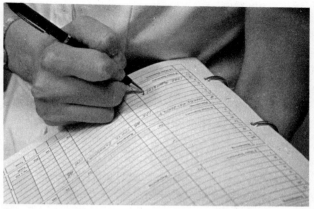

Figure 11-5. Charting.

Hickman, Broviac, and Groshong Catheters

1. Dressing and site care is usually done three times a week if the patient is stable or at home, daily for immunocompromised or postoperative patients (Schwartz-Fulton and Tischenko, 1985)
2. Sterile dressings can include traditional gauze or transparent dressings (Carelli and Herink, 1984).
3. Some institutions suggest that the nurse wear a mask during site care and dressing change, especially when caring for patients who are immunocompromised.
4. An example of a procedure for site care and dressing change follows:
   - Follow strict aseptic technique.
   - Wash hands with antiseptic soap.
   - Assemble necessary equipment.
   - Put on sterile gloves.
   - Remove old dressing and inspect site for any signs of infection.
   Erythema
   Swelling
   Serous, serosanguineous, or purulent drainage
   - Dispose of contaminated gloves and supplies.

- Wash hands.
- Put on sterile gloves.
- Clean the catheter exit site with a hydrogen peroxide–soaked swab to remove any crusting.
- Dry the site and surrounding area as needed with a sterile swab.
- Starting at the catheter exit site and moving about 2 inches from the exit site outward, clean the skin area with an antiseptic solution (povidone-iodine swabs generally are used) and allow the solution to remain on the skin for at least 60 seconds; then pat dry with sterile gauze.
- Prepare the proximal 3 inches of the catheter with the antiseptic solution.
- Apply antiseptic ointment (povidone-iodine generally is used) to the catheter exit site if desired. (This step is usually omitted if a transparent dressing is used.)
- Cover the catheter exit site with sterile dressing.
- Coil tubing over dressing and tape.

Implantable Venous Access Ports
1. Since these devices are totally subcutaneous, no site care techniques or dressing changes are needed.

Catheter Maintenance
Peripheral Catheters
(See Chapter 6 for maintaining the peripheral catheter.)

Central Venous Catheters
1. Administration sets should be changed every 24 to 48 hours.
2. The use of a $0.2\text{-}\mu$ air-eliminating filter is recommended (NITA, 1982).
   - Fat emulsions should not be filtered.
3. Precautions against air embolism must be taken during set change and all other catheter manipulations
   - Place the patient in the supine position.

- Have the patient perform the Valsalva maneuver.
- Secure all tubing junctions with tape or Luer lock connectors.
- Use air-eliminating filters when possible.

4. Parenteral nutrition lines are to be considered inviolate and dedicated to the parenteral nutrition solution; draw blood and give other infusions peripherally or through another lumen on multilumen catheters.

5. Never add on any in-line devices such as stopcocks or burettes to the parenteral nutrition line.

6. Flush central venous catheters with 1 ml to 3 ml of heparinized saline (100 units/ml) every 8 hours if used as intermittent infusion devices.

7. Before and after the administration of infusion through the catheter, flush the lumen with 3 ml to 5 ml of sterile normal saline (use 10 ml if solution is blood or if blood is drawn from the catheter); then flush with heparinized saline.

8. If catheters are used as intermittent infusion devices, change the injection cap once a week or as institutional policy dictates.

Hickman and Broviac Catheters

1. When used for continuous infusion, the IV solution and tubing (and filter, if used) should be routinely changed every 24 to 48 hours according to institutional policy (Simmons, 1982; NITA, 1982).

2. An example of a procedure for changing the administration set during continuous infusion follows:
   - Follow strict aseptic technique.
   - Wash hands with soap and water.
   - Put on sterile gloves.
   - Clean the junction and the hub of the catheter with alcohol swabsticks, being especially careful not to touch the catheter–IV tubing junction.
   - Clamp the catheter carefully using a rubber-shod clamp.
   - Immediately turn off the outdated infusion. (Clamping the catheter while the solution is still

infusing helps to prevent backflow of blood into the catheter lumen.)
- Remove the outdated tubing and gently insert the sterile Luer tip of the new tubing into the catheter hub.
- Turn the infusion on and immediately remove the rubber-shod clamp.
- Tape the catheter–IV tubing junction securely.

3. If used for intermittent infusion administration, the catheter must be flushed with heparinized saline after administration of the intermittent IV solution or medication, after transfusion or withdrawal of blood, before a Luer lock cap is attached, and daily when the catheter is not used for infusion.

4. An example of a procedure for flushing the catheter during intermittent infusion follows:
- Follow strict aseptic technique.
- Wash hands with soap and water.
- Draw 2.5 ml heparinized saline (10–100 units of heparin per milliliter) into a syringe (Pituk et al, 1983).
- Clamp the catheter carefully using a rubber-shod clamp.
- Put on sterile gloves.
- Clean the top of the Luer lock injection cap with alcohol wipe or povidone-iodine.
- Insert the needle of the syringe containing heparinized saline through the injection cap.
- Release the catheter clamp.
- Irrigate the catheter with heparin solution (irrigate to flush line thoroughly).
- Clamp the catheter during injection, leaving last 0.5 ml of heparin solution in the syringe. (This prevents backflow of blood and clot formation.)
- Remove the needle and syringe from the injection port.
- Tape the injection cap securely.
- Change the injection cap once each week or when needed.

Groshong Catheter

1. When used for continuous infusion, the IV solution and tubing (and filter, if used) should be routinely changed every 24 to 48 hours according to institutional policy (Simmons, 1982; NITA, 1982).
2. Because of its unique two-way valve design, the Groshong catheter requires no clamping or heparin flushing.
3. A 5-ml saline flush after each administration or once a week maintains catheter patency; a 20-ml saline flush is recommended after infusion or withdrawal of blood (Rosenblum, 1986).

Implantable Venous Access Ports

1. An example of a procedure to access the port follows:
   - Follow strict aseptic technique.
   - Wash hands with soap and water.
   - Put on sterile gloves.
   - Palpate the skin over the port to identify its contours and establish anatomical landmarks.
   - Stabilize the port and palpate the port septum.
   - Using a circular scrubbing motion, clean the skin over and around the port three times with antiseptic solution (povidone-iodine swabs generally are used), and allow the solution to air dry (Schulmeister, 1987).
   - Using only a special Huber point needle (22-gauge straight needle for bolus injections; 22-gauge 90-degree-angle needle for continuous infusions), slowly insert the needle through the skin into the center of the septum until the back of the portal is felt; a local anesthetic may be used to decrease the pain of needle insertion (0.1 ml–0.15 ml of lidocaine 2%).
2. For bolus injection, using a straight 22-gauge Huber needle, flush the port with 3 ml of saline before injection of the drug (if no swelling after the saline flush, the needle is considered to be patent); give the drug injection, then flush the port with 3 ml to 5 ml normal

saline, followed by 3 ml of heparinized saline (100 units/ml).

- Following aspiration of a blood sample, flush the catheter with 20 ml of saline to ensure complete removal of blood from the port.
- To remove the Huber needle from the port, stabilize the port between two fingers and gently pull the needle out while maintaining slight positive pressure on the syringe.
- During injection of any medication, observe the site carefully for signs of extravasation, such as leakage or swelling, and be alert to patient's complaints of burning or pain at the site.

3. For continuous infusion, a 90-degree 22-gauge Huber point needle is inserted into the port, secured with tape, and covered with a sterile transparent dressing.

- Begin the continuous infusion at the prescribed rate; an infusion pump can be used according to the port manufacturer's directions.
- Inspect the site at least every 8 hours, hourly if a vesicant infusion is being given.
- Change the tubing at least every 48 hours.
- Change the transparent dressing every 3 to 5 days.
- The needle can remain in place for up to 7 days (Speciale, 1985; Joseph, 1987); if the infusion lasts for longer than 7 days, a new needle should be inserted.
- At the completion of the continuous infusion, the port is flushed with heparinized saline (100 units/ml) and the Huber needle is removed.

4. These ports should be vigorously flushed with heparinized saline every 28 days to maintain patency if not used within that period.

Solution Delivery

1. All parenteral nutrition solutions should be prepared aseptically and refrigerated until just before use.

2. Each bag or bottle should be labeled with an expiration date and time.
3. No solution should be allowed to hang for longer than 24 hours.
4. Solution containers should be examined for integrity, and contents should be inspected for any signs of particulate matter or turbidity suggestive of contamination.
5. No additions should be made to the solution once it has left the pharmacy; if adjustments must be made, the solution should be sent back to the pharmacy for correction.
6. The physician usually orders a gradual initiation of the solution to allow the pancreas time to adjust to large glucose loads.
   - The initial rate is usually 60 ml to 80 ml/hr the first 24 hours.
   - There is a gradual increase of approximately 20-ml/hr every 24 to 48 hours.
7. Flow rates of the solution must be maintained at prescribed levels to prevent such complications as hyperglycemia or hypoglycemia.
8. Infusion devices may be used to ensure safe delivery of the parenteral nutrition solution, with volumetric pumps being preferred over controllers for greater accuracy.

Monitoring Parenteral Nutrition Therapy

1. After initiation of parenteral nutrition therapy, the patient should be monitored closely.
   - Check temperature and vital signs every 6 hours.
   - Monitor urine sugars every 6 hours and alert the physician if $>2^+$
   - Perform daily blood glucose determinations.
   - Maintain I and O (intake and output) records.
   - Check daily weight.

2. Once blood glucose has remained stable for several days, blood glucose can be monitored twice a week.
3. Other laboratory parameters should be checked twice a week:
   - Liver function tests
   - Electrolyte profiles
   - Blood urea nitrogen (BUN) and creatinine
   - Other tests as ordered
4. Nitrogen balance studies may be done to evaluate effectiveness of therapy.
5. There should be constant vigilance for signs of septic complications:
   - Increase in patient's temperature
   - Sudden "spilling" of sugar in the urine
   - Erythema, swelling, tenderness, or drainage at the insertion site
6. Provide excellent oral care.
   - Flavored mouthwashes
   - Lip balms

Termination of Parenteral Nutrition Therapy

1. As with initiation, the physician usually prescribes gradual termination of parenteral nutrition therapy.
2. Decreasing the solution amount by 1 liter/day will usually prevent rebound hypoglycemia.
3. Before termination, arrange for an alternate form of nutritional support.
4. An example of procedure for catheter removal follows:
   - Follow strict aseptic technique.
   - Wash hands with antiseptic soap.
   - Put on sterile gloves.
   - Remove dressing over site.
   - Remove suture if present.
   - Instruct the patient to perform the Valsalva maneuver.
   - Using a gentle but continuous pulling motion, re-

move the catheter. (For catheters such as the Hickman that contain a Dacron cuff, blunt dissection of the cuff from the subcutaneous tissues may be necessary; catheters such as the implantable venous access ports must be removed surgically.)
· Measure and inspect the catheter—make sure it is intact.
· Clean area with an antiseptic solution.
· Consider applying antiseptic ointment.
· Apply pressure dressing.
· Dispose of contaminated gloves and supplies.
· Chart.

Bibliography

American Medical Association: Guidelines for essential trace element preparations for parenteral use: A statement by the Nutrition Advisory Group. JPEN 3:263, 1979

American Medical Association Department of Foods and Nutrition: Multivitamin preparations for parenteral use: A statement by the Nutrition Advisory Group. JPEN 3:259, 1979

Bottino J, McCredie KB, Groschel DM, et al: Long-term intravenous therapy with peripherally inserted silicone elastomer central venous catheters in patients with malignant diseases. Cancer 43:1937, 1979

Carelli RM, Herink E: Hickman/Broviac catheters, results of survey and patient care considerations. NITA 7:287, 1984

Colley R, Appleby L, Ayello E, et al: Hyperalimentation standards of practice of the National Intravenous Therapy Association, Inc. (NITA). NITA 4:105, 1981

Foltz A: Evaluation of implanted infusion devices. NITA 10:49, 1987

Ganz NM, Presswood GM, Goldberg R et al: Effects of dressing type and change interval on intravenous therapy complication rates. Diagn Microbiol Infect Dis 2:325, 1984

Gebarski SS, Gebarski KS: Chemotherapy port "Twiddler's syndrome": A need for preinjection radiography. Cancer 54:38, 1984

Goodman SG, Wickham R: Venous access devices: An overview. Oncology Nursing Forum 11(5):16, 1984

Griggs B: A Basic Nursing Guide to Providing TPN for the Adult Patient. Monograph, ASPEN, 1984

Hardin TC: Complex parenteral nutrition solutions: I. Drug additives. Nutr Sup Serv 3:58, 1983

Joseph P: Reader questions: How long should subcutaneous I.V. devices be left in place? Hospital Infection Control, pp 27–28, February 1987

Lawson M, Kavanagh T, McCredie K et al: Comparison of transparent dressing to paper tape dressing over central venous catheter sites. NITA 9:40, 1986

Linder LE: Material thrombogenicity in central venous catheterization. JPEN pp 399–406, July/Aug 1984

Lokich J, Bothe A, Benotti P, et al: Complications and management of implanted venous access catheters. J Clin Oncol 3(5):710, 1985

Maki D, Will L: Colonization and infection associated with transparent dressings for central venous catheters—a comparative trial. Presented at Association for Practitioners in Infection Control, National Meeting, Washington, DC, June 1984

National Intravenous Therapy Association: Standards of Practice. NITA 5:19, 1982

Pestana C: Fluids and Electrolytes in the Surgical Patient, 3rd ed. Baltimore, Williams & Wilkins, 1985

Pituk TL, DeYoung JL, Levin HJ: Volumes of selected central venous catheters and implications for heparin flush use. NITA 6:98, 1983

Powell C, Regan C, Fabri P et al: Evaluation of Op-Site catheter dressings for parenteral nutrition: A prospective, randomized study. JPEN 6:143, 1982

Rosenblum B: Long-term venous access for home infusion therapy. Infusion 10(2):39, 1986

Schulmeister L: A comparison of skin preparation procedures for accessing implanted ports. NITA 10:45, 1987

Schwartz-Fulton J, Colley R, Valanis B et al: Hyperalimentation dressings and skin flora. NITA 4:354, 1981

Schwartz-Fulton J, Tischenko MM: Hickman catheter exit site

skin sensitivities in an oncology patient population. NITA 8:63, 1985

Simmons BP: Guidelines for the prevention of intravascular infections. From: Centers for Disease Control. Guidelines for the Prevention and Control of Nosocomial Infections. NITA 5:40, 1982

Speciale JL: Infuse-A-Port, a new path for I.V. chemotherapy. Nursing85, pp 40–43, October 1985

Woolfson AMJ, Heatley RV, Allison SP: Insulin to inhibit protein catabolism after injury. N Engl J Med 300:14, 1979

12 ▷ Complications of Parenteral Nutrition

Key Points

1. Mechanical complications
2. Septic complications
3. Metabolic complications
4. Psychosocial complications

Mechanical Complications

Pneumothorax, Hemothorax, Chylothorax, Hydrothorax

Description

Air, blood, lymph, or infusion fluid collects in the pleural cavity owing to pleura, vein, or thoracic duct injury during catheter placement.

Assessment

Sharp chest pain or decreased breath sounds may be present, or radiographic evidence may be seen; thoracentesis can confirm the diagnosis. Vital signs and respiratory status should be continually monitored.

Nursing Interventions

1. Provide appropriate nursing care of the chest tube if one was placed.
2. Extreme care must be used during catheter placement; only well-trained and experienced nurses should assist the physician during catheterization.

Catheter Malposition

Description
The needle or introducer slips out of the vein during catheter placement.

Assessment
The first sign is catheter passage becomes difficult or impossible during placement; later, cardiac arrhythmias can occur. Difficulties and irregularities can occur in the flow of infusate.

Nursing Interventions
1. Monitor fluid flow and patient response (including cardiac rhythm) during infusion.
2. Advise the physician if irregularities occur.
3. Support and assess the patient as the physician repositions the catheter.

Pericardial Tamponade

Description
The atrium is penetrated by the catheter.

Assessment
Cardiovascular collapse with neck vein distention, a narrow pulse pressure, and hypotension, with or without symptoms of congestive heart failure, can suggest the possibility of pericardial tamponade.

Nursing Interventions
1. Emergency treatment by the physician is critical; it usually involves aspiration of the pericardial sac.
2. The causative catheter should be withdrawn and replaced following resuscitation.
3. Use of highly beveled rigid catheters should be discouraged.
4. Provide continuous assessment of patient status and participate in emergency procedures appropriate to the nurse's role.

Brachial Plexus or Phrenic Nerve Injury

Description
The brachial plexus nerve network or phrenic nerve is injured during catheter placement.

Assessment
There may be a tingling sensation in the fingers, pain shooting down the arm, or paralysis of the arms.

Nursing Interventions
1. Treatment is symptomatic and may not always resolve the injury.
2. Physical therapy may be indicated for paralysis.

Subclavian Artery Laceration

Description
The subclavian artery is accidentally lacerated during an attempt to find the subclavian vein.

Assessment
A pulsating wave of bright red arterial blood fills the syringe during catheter placement; blood spurts forth if the syringe is disconnected from the needle.

Nursing Interventions
1. Apply direct pressure on the artery for 10 minutes.
2. If patient's clotting times are prolonged, apply direct pressure on the artery for 30 minutes.

Air Embolism

Description
There is passage of air into the heart with the result of an intracardiac air lock at the pulmonic valve, preventing ejection of blood from the right side of the heart.

Assessment
Signs and symptoms may vary with the severity of the air embolism and may include dyspnea, apnea, hypoxia, dis-

orientation, tachycardia, hypotension, or a precordial murmur.

Nursing Interventions
1. The patient should be placed in the left lateral Trendelenburg position.
2. Direct intracardiac needle aspiration of the air may be done by the physician.
3. To prevent air embolism, precautions must be taken during catheter placement, tubing changes, and catheter removal.
4. All tubing junctions should be properly secured.

Catheter Embolism

Description
The sheared off or broken part of a catheter becomes lodged in the great veins, the right side of the heart, or the pulmonary outflow tract.

Assessment
This complication is usually suspected when the catheter is removed and it appears shortened or sheared off.

Nursing Interventions
1. Immediately obtain an x-ray film and decrease patient mobility.
2. In many instances the catheter may be spotted and retrieved with a specially designed snare that is guided under fluoroscopic control.
3. In some cases a thoracotomy may be performed by the physician.

Great-Vein Thrombosis

Description
There is thrombosis of the superior vena cava or its tributaries caused by long-term central catheterization. Pulmonary emboli are often secondary to great-vein thromboses.

Assessment

Recognition is often impeded by variability of presentation: there may be no symptoms, arm and neck pain may present, or signs and symptoms of pulmonary embolus may present.

Nursing Intervention

1. Preventive measures include the use of silicone elastomer catheters, which are reported to cause fewer incidences of fibrin sheath formation, and the addition of 1000 units/liter of heparin to the infusate to prevent thrombosis.
2. Thrombolytic therapy has recently been shown to be of benefit. (Refer to the nursing interventions in Chapter 8, the section Needle/Cannula Occlusion.)

Catheter Occlusion

Description

The catheter becomes occluded owing to fibrin sheath formation over the tip.

Assessment

The flow of infusion is slowed or stopped completely. All IV tubing should be checked for kinks or obstructions; electronic infusion devices should be checked for malfunction; and the integrity of the in-line filter must be checked (if it is being used) to rule out other potential causes of the occlusion.

Nursing Interventions

1. Patency can usually be restored by a small dose of streptokinase. (Refer to the nursing interventions in Chapter 8, the section Needle/Cannula Occlusion.)

Leaking Catheter

Description

A small puncture in the catheter causes a leak that slowly saturates the dressing over the insertion site; leaks could also be due to a break in one of the components of the IV tubing or a separation at a junction or connector.

Assessment

Usually a saturated dressing is the first evidence of a leak.

Nursing Interventions

1. Check all tubing connections and junctions to make sure they are properly seated.
2. Use of Luer lock connectors is recommended.
3. If it is found that the catheter itself is the cause of the leak, it must be removed or aseptically repaired.

Septic Complications

Local Infection at Catheter Entry Site

Description

A local infection at the site of catheter insertion is usually caused by organisms improperly removed from the hands of personnel or the skin of patients before catheter insertion or manipulation is performed.

Assessment

Erythema, swelling, drainage, or pain is present at the catheter entry site; a rise in the patient's temperature may occur.

Nursing Interventions

1. Treatment may include catheter removal or administration of appropriate antibiotics, as ordered by the physician, with the catheter left in place.
2. The key to prevention is strict adherence to infection control procedures including scrupulous handwashing practices, proper skin preparation before catheter insertion or manipulation, proper site care and dressing change protocols, and extreme care in the handling of any parenteral nutrition equipment or infusate.

Catheter Sepsis

Description

The usual cause is contamination of the catheter entry site, whereby organisms (usually from hands of personnel caring for the catheter) grow and migrate along the catheter, infecting it or its fibrin sheath; hematogenous seeding of the whole system can then occur, leading to septic complications.

Assessment

Any elevation in temperature should be a warning; sudden "spilling" of sugar in the urine may also be an indication of impending sepsis. Previous local site infection can progress to sepsis.

Nursing Interventions

1. Immediately notify the physician when fever presents.
2. Blood cultures may be ordered.
3. The physician may decide to remove the catheter, and semiquantitative culture of the catheter tip should be done (Maki et al, 1977).
4. Appropriate antibiotics are usually prescribed by the physician.
5. The key to prevention is strict adherence to infection control procedures including scrupulous handwashing practices, proper skin preparation before catheter insertion or manipulation, proper site care and dressing change protocols, and extreme care in the handling of any parenteral nutrition equipment or infusate.

Metabolic Complications

Hyperglycemia

Description

There is a rapid rise in serum glucose level beyond the ability of the pancreas to secrete insulin to handle it.

Assessment

The first sign is usually glycosuria, which may be followed by nausea, vomiting, headaches, and lethargy; serum glucose levels are usually greater than 200 mg/dl.

Nursing Interventions

1. Hyperglycemia should be prevented by adjustment of the infusion rate and, subsequently, the amount of glucose released to the blood.
2. The addition of insulin to the infusion as ordered by the physician may be necessary in some patients to maintain blood glucose levels below 200 mg/dl.

Hyperosmolar Hyperglycemic Nonketotic Dehydration (HHNK)

Description

HHNK is a syndrome characterized by hyperglycemia and dehydration with hyperosmolarity and azotemia, but not ketosis. This is in contrast to diabetic ketoacidosis, which has the presence of ketones in the urine and breath and metabolic acidosis.

Assessment

Identifying patients with HHNK can sometimes be difficult; clinical findings are those of confusion, neurologic dysfunction that may progress to coma, and dehydration. Laboratory data pointing to HHNK include the following:

- Serum osmolality over 300 mOsm/kg
- Serum glucose levels of 200 mg to 1000 mg/dl
- Serum sodium greater than 150 mEq/liter

Nursing Interventions

1. Treatment usually consists in fluid replacement, insulin administration, and cessation of the hypertonic glucose solution as ordered by the physician.
2. Monitor patient weight and fluid balance (intake and output records).
3. Monitor clinical signs of hypotension, tachycardia, and oliguria.

Hypoglycemia

Description
Serum glucose drops following an abrupt decrease in the infusion rate of hypertonic glucose solution.

Assessment
The serum glucose value is less than 50 mg/dl. The patient may complain of weakness; headache; chills; tingling in the extremities or mouth; cold, clammy skin; thirst; hunger; or apprehension. Other symptoms may include diaphoresis, decreased levels of consciousness, and changes in vital signs.

Nursing Interventions
1. Prevention is accomplished by decreasing hypertonic glucose solutions slowly.
2. Before the patient resumes oral nutrition the rate of infusion of glucose should slow by approximately 20 ml/hr/day to a rate of 60 ml/hr as the patient begins oral intake.

Essential Fatty Acid Deficiency (EFAD)

Description
Signs and symptoms are due to the cessation of fat intake, depriving the patient of at least one fatty acid, linoleic, that cannot be synthesized by humans.

Assessment
Signs and symptoms can include alopecia, brittle nails, desquamating dermatitis, delayed wound healing, decreased immune function, thrombocytopenia, and fatty infiltration of the liver.

Nursing Interventions
1. Clinical symptoms of EFAD reverse on administration of linoleic acid; the following three treatments are now recommended:
    - Oral administration of 15 ml of safflower oil three

times a day if the patient can tolerate fluids by mouth
- Topical application of the oil (15 ml) three times a day to allow for absorption through the skin
- IV lipid infusion in amounts of 4% to 10% of total calories every day; can be given as 500 ml of 10% or 20% fat emulsion two or three times a week

Electrolyte Imbalances

Description
Electrolyte imbalances usually occur in parenteral nutrition as hypostates and hyperstates of sodium and potassium, hypophosphatemia, and hypomagnesemia.

Assessment
Signs and symptoms of electrolyte imbalance vary according to the individual electrolyte (see Tables 1-3 to 1-10 in Chapter 1 for further information).

Nursing Interventions
1. Monitor laboratory values and adjust parenteral nutrition solutions as ordered by the physician.

Vitamin and Trace Element Deficiencies

Description
Nutritional requirements for vitamins and trace elements have been under investigation for only approximately 10 years. (Refer to the AMA guidelines for the daily administration of IV vitamins and trace elements, in Chapter 11.)

Assessment
A variety of signs and symptoms are possible with vitamin or trace element deficiencies, including anemia states, retarded growth, weight loss, abnormal glucose tolerance, nausea and vomiting, changes in skin and hair, skeletal abnormalities, muscle soreness, weak nails, hair loss, mental depression, and impaired healing abilities.

Nursing Interventions
1. Monitor patients for signs of possible vitamin or trace element deficiencies.
2. Monitor laboratory test results.
3. Adjust parenteral nutrition solutions as ordered by the physician.

Psychosocial Complications

Psychosocial Adjustments to Therapy

Description
There is difficulty in coping with anxiety and stress related to the meaning of long-term therapy, alteration of body image, changes in level of activity, and inability to eat.

Assessment
A thorough evaluation of psychosocial aspects is important, with continual reassessment as treatment progresses.

Nursing Interventions
1. Encourage patients and family members to participate in self-help groups or other social groups.
2. Be available to answer patient's and family members' questions concerning therapy.
3. Encourage family members to help with the patient's care.
4. Encourage honest expression of feelings.
5. Promote independent decision making when appropriate.

Bibliography

Appleby L: Initiation, maintenance, and termination of total parenteral nutrition. NITA 6:31, 1983

Bjornson HS, Colley R, Bower RH et al: Association between the number of microorganisms present at the catheter insertion site and the colonization of the central venous catheter in patients receiving total parenteral venous nutrition. Surgery 94:720, 1982

Bower RH: Metabolic complications of parenteral nutrition therapy. NITA 6:37, 1983

Estner MJ, Goldfarb IW, Savini MJ et al: Internal jugular vein thrombosis: A rare complication of long-term indwelling subclavian vein catheters. NITA 9:220, 1986

Fabri PJ, Mirtallo JM, Ruberg RL et al: Incidence and prevention of thrombosis of the subclavian vein during total parenteral nutrition. Surg Gynecol Obstet 155:238, 1982

Hennessy K: HHNK dehydration. Am J Nurs, pp 1425–1426, October 1983

Hurtubise MR, Bottino JC, Lawson M et al: Restoring patency of occluded central venous catheters. Arch Surg 115:212, 1980

Lokich JL, Becker B: Subclavian vein thrombosis in patients treated with infusion chemotherapy for advanced malignancy. Cancer 52:1586, 1983

Maki DG, Weise CE, Sarafin HW: A semiquantitative culture method for identifying intravenous catheter-related infection. N Engl J Med 296:1305, 1977

Plumer AL, Colley R, Duty VP: Total parenteral nutrition—nursing practice: Psychological Aspects. In Principles and Practice of Intravenous Therapy, 3rd ed. Boston, Little, Brown Co, 1982

Ross AH, Griffith CD, Anderson JR et al: Thromboembolic complications with silicone elastomer subclavian catheters. JPEN 6:61, 1982

Ryan JA Jr, Abel RM, Abbott WM et al: Catheter complications in total parenteral nutrition. N Engl J Med 290:757, 1974

Ryan JA Jr, Gough J: Complication of central venous catheterization for total parenteral nutrition: The role of the nurse. NITA 7:29, 1984

Schneider PJ: Hyperosmolar coma: A serious complication in TPN patients. Infusion 9:141, 1985

Unit V

Special Topics

13 ▷ Hemodynamic Monitoring

Key Points

1. Central lines
2. Arterial catheters
3. Pulmonary artery catheters

Central Lines

Central venous pressure (CVP) measurements can be determined by using a manometer that is connected to a central venous catheter. These catheters are usually placed in or near the right atrium by access through the subclavian, basilic, or jugular vein. CVP readings help to do the following:

1. Assess the capacity of the right side of the heart to receive and eject blood
2. Monitor fluid replacement
3. Evaluate blood volume

Description of the System

1. See Chapter 11 for procedures involving insertion of a central line and site care recommendations.
2. A disposable CVP manometer containing stopcock, extension tubing, and leveling device is connected to an IV pole.
3. The manometer and extension tubing are filled with the prescribed IV fluid.
4. The extension tubing is connected to the patient's catheter and the infusion rate is regulated.

5. The position of the manometer is adjusted so that the stopcock aligns horizontally with the patient's right atrium, and the leveling device of the manometer is centered.
6. The stopcock is turned to the container-to-manometer position so that the manometer fills with IV fluid; the stopcock is then turned to the manometer-to-patient position.
7. After the fluid column stabilizes and the manometer is lightly tapped to dislodge air bubbles, the CVP reading is taken from the lowest level that the fluid reaches, as read from the bottom of the meniscus.
8. The stopcock is returned to the container-to-patient position, all connections are secured, and the IV fluid rate is adjusted.

Special Considerations

1. Hospital personnel should wash their hands before manipulating any part of the CVP system or the central venous line.
2. CVP is usually measured at 15-, 30-, and 60-minute intervals; if the patient's readings deviate from the prescribed CVP range, alert the physician.
3. The average CVP range is between 5 and 15 cm H_2O, but this can vary from patient to patient.
4. If the patient is connected to a ventilator and is receiving positive end-expiratory pressure (PEEP), the CVP readings will tend to be higher; make sure all subsequent readings from that patient are taken while the patient is on the ventilator.
5. Falsely low results may be seen if the CVP reading is taken while the patient is sitting up.
6. When taking a reading, the fluid level in the manometer should fluctuate slightly as the patient breathes; if this fluctuation does not occur, it may mean the catheter tip is pressed against the wall of the vein; ask the patient to cough—this will usually reposition the catheter.

Arterial Catheters

The function of the cardiovascular system is to carry oxygen and nutrients to cells and to remove metabolic wastes from cells for excretion. Accomplishing these tasks is the result of a complex interplay between the heart, the blood vessels, and the blood itself. It is easy to see that hemodynamic monitoring of the arterial system, as well as the venous system just discussed, is essential to measuring the effectiveness of the cardiovascular system.

An indwelling arterial catheter allows for the following:

1. Continuous and accurate arterial pressure readings
2. Assessment of the cardiovascular effects of vasoactive drugs
3. Drawing of arterial blood for arterial blood gas determinations

Arterial catheters are usually inserted into the brachial, the radial, or, occasionally, the femoral artery. The catheter is connected to an electronic pressure transducer that converts fluid pressure into electronic signals that can be displayed on a monitor and also recorded on paper tape. A visible and audible alarm can be set to respond if pressure exceeds preset limits. The patency of the line is usually maintained by a closed continuous flush system of heparinized saline administered under pressure to reduce the risk of clot formation.

Description of the System

1. A 500-ml bag of heparinized saline (1–2 units of heparin per milliliter of 0.9% sodium chloride) is connected to a nonvented administration set containing a microdrop chamber.
2. The heparinized saline bag is placed inside a pressure infusor bag.
3. The administration set is connected by high-pressure tubing to a disposable transducer dome that contains

a continuous flush device and several three-way stop-cocks.

4. After the system is flushed with the heparinized solution, all air bubbles are removed and all connections are secured, and the dome is attached to the transducer.

5. The transducer is then mounted on an IV pole at the level of the patient's right atrium.

Catheter Insertion and Site Care

1. Strict aseptic technique must be followed by everyone involved in manipulating any portion of the pressure monitoring system; handwashing with an antiseptic soap should be performed by all personnel.

2. The physician will perform the catheter insertion, with assistance from the nurse; sterile gloves should be worn by the physician during the insertion procedure.

3. The insertion site is carefully prepared with 1% to 2% tincture of iodine or povidone-iodine.

4. The physician will insert the 19- or 20-gauge Teflon catheter percutaneously, if possible, or by surgical cutdown if necessary.

5. After insertion, the catheter is firmly anchored and a topical antiseptic ointment (povidone-iodine ointment generally is used) is applied to the site, which is then covered with a sterile occlusive dressing.

6. Patency of the line is maintained by infusion of the heparinized saline solution at a rate of 3 ml/hr through the continuous flush device.

7. The patient should be evaluated at least once a day for evidence of any catheter-related complications; this evaluation should include gentle palpation of the insertion site through the intact dressing, with visual site inspection if the patient has unexplained fever or tenderness/pain at the site.

8. If no complications occur, the catheter can be left in place for up to 4 days.

9. The sterile dressing should be changed at least every 48 hours, and the antiseptic ointment reapplied if used.

10. The container of flush solution should be changed every 24 hours.

11. The chamber dome, administration tubing, and continuous flow device should be replaced every 48 hours.

12. Follow specific instructions from the manufacturer on calibration and use of the monitoring equipment.

Special Considerations

1. The pressure monitoring system should be kept as simple as possible, avoiding unnecessary tubing, stopcocks, and connectors; minimize manipulation of the system, and when possible limit the number of times the closed system must be entered.

2. Eliminate the stagnant fluid column associated with a "side spur" of IV tubing.

3. Maintain physical separation of the transducer from the port used for routine blood sampling.

4. Disposable transducer domes or other disposable components should not be resterilized or reused.

5. The space between the transducer head and the disposable dome membrane should be left dry, or the space should be filled with normal saline, bacteriostatic water, or 70% alcohol but *not* a glucose-containing solution, since glucose-containing solutions can support the growth of microorganisms.

6. Transducers should be cleaned with hydrogen peroxide and then sterilized with ethylene oxide between uses and should be stored in such a way as to prevent contamination before use on the next patient.

7. Take meticulous care of the stopcock port by replacing sterile caps after each manipulation, cleaning the port with povidone-iodine or alcohol, or covering the port with an injection cap through which blood could be drawn after surface sterilization.

8. Change the stopcock segment routinely.

Arterial Blood Sample Aspiration
From the Arterial Catheter

1. Whenever possible, reduce the risk of contamination by limiting the number of aspirations to avoid unnecessary opening of the closed system.
2. Wash hands with an antibacterial soap.
3. Heparinize a 10-ml glass syringe:
   - Draw 1 ml of aqueous heparin (1 : 1000) into the glass syringe through a 20-gauge needle.
   - Rotate the barrel of the syringe while pulling the plunger back to approximately the 7-ml mark to allow the heparin to coat the inside of the surface of the syringe.
   - Expel the heparin from the syringe.
4. Put on sterile gloves.
5. Flush the arterial line by activating the fast-flush release on the continuous flush device.
6. Attach a 5-ml nonheparinized syringe to the stopcock port, open the stopcock to release arterial blood flow, and gently aspirate 5 ml of blood.
7. Shut off arterial blood flow and remove and discard this syringe.
8. Remove the needle from the heparinized glass syringe and discard it; attach the syringe to the port, open the stopcock to release arterial blood, and allow the syringe to fill with 3 ml to 5 ml of blood.
9. Shut off arterial blood flow, remove the syringe, place a rubber cap on the tip of the syringe, and place the syringe in an ice bath for immediate transport to the laboratory.
10. Clear the blood from the sampling port by using the fast-flush release of the continuous flush device.
11. Recap the stopcock port with a sterile cap, and flush the line completely using the fast-flush release.

Pulmonary Artery Catheters

Pulmonary artery catheters are multilumen, balloon-tipped, flow-directed catheters inserted percutaneously into the subclavian, jugular, or femoral vein, or by a venous cutdown in the antecubital fossa. As the catheter is threaded into the vein and the tip passes the superior vena cava, the balloon is inflated and the venous circulation carries the catheter tip through the right atrium and the tricuspid valve; it then enters the right ventricle and passes on into a branch of the pulmonary artery, where it becomes wedged in one of the smaller vessels. The balloon is then deflated and the catheter tip comes to rest in the pulmonary artery. The catheter is connected to a pressure transducer and various monitors, and it can be used to do the following:

1. Measure pulmonary artery pressure (PAP)
2. Measure pulmonary capillary wedge pressure (PCWP)
3. Measure CVP
4. Administer IV fluids
5. Obtain blood samples
6. Detect complications of acute myocardial infarction
7. Evaluate the effects of certain drugs
8. Assess vascular volume

Description of the System and Its Functions

1. Pulmonary artery catheters (*e.g.*, the Swan-Ganz catheter manufactured by Edwards Laboratories) typically have four or five lumina (Fig. 13-1); examples of lumen functions follow:
   - Distal lumen. Used to measure PAP and PCWP and to obtain mixed venous blood samples for oxygen-saturation determinations
   - Inflation lumen. Used to inflate the balloon at the tip of the catheter during PCWP determination
   - Thermistor lumen. Contains two fine wires leading to a thermistor, which measures the patient's cardiac output
   - Proximal lumen. Opens into the right atrium where it can be used to measure CVP and to infuse IV solutions

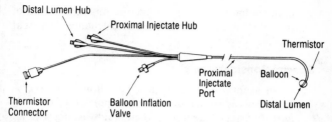

Figure 13-1. Swan-Ganz® thermodilution catheter (Model 93A-131-7F) (Courtesy of American Edwards Laboratories, Division of American Hospital Supply Corporation, Santa Ana, CA).

2. Equipment for the system consists of the catheter, a 500-ml bag of heparinized saline (1–2 units of heparin per milliliter of 0.9% sodium chloride), a pressure cuff, a nonvented administration set with microdrip chamber, 3 to 4 feet of pressure tubing, a continuous-flush device, a transducer and disposable transducer dome, high-pressure extension tubing, a three-way stopcock, a transducer cable, and various monitors.

3. The physician will perform the catheter insertion, with assistance from the nurse; sterile gloves should be worn by the physician during the insertion procedure. (See Chapter 11 for procedures involving insertion of a central line and site care recommendations.)

4. PAP can be determined by recording pulmonary artery systolic pressure (PAS), pulmonary artery diastolic pressure (PAD), and mean pressure values.

5. PCWP can be determined by inflating the balloon of the catheter and measuring the pressure obtained distal to the branch of the pulmonary artery that has been occluded by the balloon.

6. Cardiac output can be determined indirectly by the thermodilution technique: a small known amount of 5% dextrose in water is injected into the right atrium by way of the proximal port of the catheter; the change in the temperature is monitored downstream

in the pulmonary artery by the thermistor in the tip of the catheter, and a minicomputer calculates the actual cardiac output.

Special Considerations

1. Strict aseptic technique must be followed by everyone involved in manipulating any portion of the pulmonary artery catheter system; handwashing with an antiseptic soap should be performed by all personnel.
2. The catheter system should be kept as simple as possible, avoiding unnecessary tubing, stopcocks, and connectors; minimize manipulation of the system, and when possible limit the number of times the closed system must be entered.
3. Patients receiving positive-pressure ventilation may have altered readings. Record all pressures while the patient is on the ventilator.
4. When measuring PCWP, do not leave the balloon inflated for longer than 1 to 2 minutes; do not introduce air into the balloon if it is suspected that the balloon has ruptured.

Bibliography

Band JD, Maki DG: Infections caused by arterial catheters used for hemodynamic monitoring. Am J Med 67:735, 1979

Bond G, Caldwell J: Septicemia from an unexpected source. RN, pp 48–49, July 1982

Bustin D: Hemodynamic Monitoring for Critical Care. Norwalk, CN, Appleton-Century-Crofts, 1986

Buxton AE, Anderson RL, Klimek J et al: Failure of disposable domes to prevent septicemia acquired from contaminated pressure transducers. Chest 74:508, 1978

Cleary TJ, MacIntyre DS, Castro M: *Serratia marcescens* bacteremias in an intensive care unit. Am J Infect Control 9:107, 1981

Donowitz LG, Marsik FJ, Hoyt JW et al: *Serratia marcescens* bacteremia from contaminated pressure transducers. JAMA 242:1749, 1979

Lantiegne KC, Civetta JM: A system for maintaining invasive pressure monitoring. Heart Lung 7:610, 1978

Maki DG, Hassemer CA: Endemic rate of fluid contamination and related septicemia in arterial pressure monitoring. Am J Med 70:733, 1981

Niemczura J: Eight rules to remember when caring for a patient with a Swan-Ganz catheter. Nursing85, pp 38–41, 1985

Plumer AL: Principles and Practice of Intravenous Therapy, 3rd ed. Boston, Little, Brown & Co, 1982

Roderick B: How to manage CVP lines. RN, pp 22–25, July 1985

Roderick MA: Infection Control in Critical Care. Rockville, Aspen Systems Corporation, 1983

Santolla A, Weckel C: A new closed system for arterial lines. RN, pp 49–52, July 1983

Scordo K: Hemodynamic monitoring: Learning to read the waves. Nursing85, pp 40–42, July 1985

Shinozaki, Deane RS, Mazuzan JE et al: Bacterial contamination of arterial lines. JAMA 249:23, 1983

Spangler RA: Update on pulmonary artery catheterization. Nursing85, pp 42–45, August 1985

Talbot GH, Skros M, Provencher M: 70% Alcohol disinfection or transducer heads: Experimental trials. Infect Control 6:237, 1985

Visalli F: The Swan-Ganz catheter. Nursing81, pp 42–47, January 1981

Walrath JM, Abbott NK, Caplan E et al: Stopcock: Bacterial contamination in invasive monitoring systems. Heart Lung 8:100, 1979

Yonkman CA, Hamory BH: Comparison of three methods of maintaining a sterile injectate system during cardiac output determinations. Am J Infect Control 12:276, 1984

14 ▷ Intravenous Drug Administration and Nursing Implications

Key Points

1. Advantages of IV route
2. Relative disadvantages of IV administration of drugs
3. Methods of IV drug administration
4. Incompatibility
5. General guidelines for nursing interventions
6. Antibiotics: Nursing implications
7. Antineoplastic agents: Nursing implications
8. Continuous narcotic infusions

Effective, safe administration of IV medications is dependent on sound knowledge of the route as well as the drugs involved. Inclusion of such content in educational programs does not ensure the existence of such knowledge (Markowitz et al, 1981). The following information is outlined to provide the framework on which to build a more extensive command of the knowledge required.

Advantages of IV Route

1. Provides for rapid absorption and, consequently, immediate action
2. Allows for continuous administration
3. Allows for uninterrupted control of rate
4. Allows for immediate termination of infusion, if indicated
5. Allows for administration of medications that are unstable when exposed to gastric juices

6. Allows for administration of medications that cannot be absorbed in the gastrointestinal tract
7. Provides route of administration in patients in whom use of the gastrointestinal tract is limited
8. Provides route of administration for medications too irritating for other routes of administration

Relative Disadvantages of IV Administration of Drugs (Leff, 1983)

1. Adsorption of drugs to materials in the IV system may lead to decreased amounts of drug actually delivered to the patient.
2. Use of more distal injection ports may result in longer onset and delayed completion time.
3. Slower flow rates may result in longer onset and completion time.
4. Larger drug dosages and slower flow rates may result in longer time for complete drug delivery.
5. Multiple drug therapy regimens may cause incompatibility problems.
6. Greater specific gravities result in a layering effect in the IV tubing, which may alter drug delivery time.
7. High osmolality and pH may cause an increased rate of phlebitis.

Methods of IV Drug Administration

Continuous Infusion

Medication is diluted in 250 ml to 1000 ml of infusate and administered over 2 to 24 hours.

Intermittent Infusion

1. IV push/IV bolus. Medication is diluted in 0.25 ml to 50 ml of infusate and infused over a 5-second to 10- to 15-minute period. Avenues of administration include venipuncture, through a primary IV line, or through an intermittent set.

2. Piggyback/add-a-line. Medication is diluted in 10 ml to 150 ml of infusate and administered over 5 minutes to 2 hours.

Syringe Pump

Medication is administered through a prefilled syringe placed in a syringe pump.

1. Advantages include the following:
   - Phlebitis may be decreased.
   - Toxicity and fluctuating blood levels are reduced.
   - Medication waste is minimized.
   - System is portable, lightweight.
   - Syringes are easily stored.
   - Equipment needed for infusion may be less costly than standard administration systems.
2. Disadvantages may include the following:
   - Prefiltering of medication may be required.
   - Orientation to use of the system is required.

Incompatibility

Definition

Incompatibility, existing when drugs cannot be combined safely or successfully, can occur between two drugs or between drug and infusate (Morris, 1979).

A clinically significant incompatibility is one that results either in a loss of the desired therapeutic effect or in new or unwanted effects.

Types

1. Therapeutic incompatibility
   - Occurs when the administration of more than one medication produces a different response in the patient than what was expected
   - Occurs when the intensity of response to the medication is altered.

2. Pharmaceutical incompatibility
   - Occurs when, as one drug is mixed with another, the physiochemical result is a product unsuitable for administration
   - May result in formation of actual precipitate, haze, gas, bubbles, or color change
   - May result in alteration of integrity and potency of the medication by a chemical reaction

Factors Affecting Compatibility/Incompatibility

- pH of the admixture
- pH of the infusate
- Type of infusate
- Additional drugs
- Buffering agents in the medications
- Preservative in the solution used for dilution
- Degree of dilution (concentration)
- Period of time the solution stands
- Order of the mixing
- Light
- Temperature

General Guidelines for Nursing Interventions

1. Review medication literature thoroughly. This material should include a complete description of materials, test conditions, and methods for drug testing; use of a stability-indicating essay method; presence of time-zero determinations; presence of replicated results; and logical conclusions flowing from the information presented (Trissel, 1985).
2. Use the expertise of the pharmacist.
3. If possible, administer only one medication in each infusate container.
4. Use freshly prepared solutions.
5. Always observe for the presence of precipitate.
   Note: The naked eye can only see precipitate greater than 50 μ in size.

6. Use final filters with additives, if not contraindicated.
7. The pH is a major key in incompatibility; usually additives are compatible if they are within the same pH range:
   - Base = 8.0–10.0
   - Acid = 3.0–5.0
8. When possible, use normal saline as a diluent, since it is more neutral and less irritating.
9. Use 50 ml to 100 ml of a diluent with antibiotics.
10. Whenever there is a question of incompatibility of fluids in the secondary set with that in the primary set, flush the system with 0.9% normal saline before and after the medication infusion.
11. Frozen parenteral products can be thawed at room temperature, in warm-water baths, or by microwave radiation.
    Note: Leaching of rubber stopper material is possible with microwave heating. Safety of microwave thawing for each parenteral product must be ascertained (Turco and Rock, 1984).
12. Promote efficient drug delivery, especially in the pediatric patient, by the following:
    - Use low-volume tubing.
    - Use the most distal injection site.
    - If the dead space at the port is large, flush the injection port following administration of the medication.
13. Assume any drug combination is incompatible until proven otherwise.
14. Since any IV medication has the potential for causing an allergic reaction, always stay with the patient for at least 5 minutes after the infusion is started for the first time.
15. After adding a drug to an IV bag, gently rotate the bag to ensure thorough mixing (Drew and Schumann, 1986).
16. If adding medication to a container that is already hung and infusing, stop the flow before injecting the additive. Following addition of the medication, gently

rotate the container to ensure mixing; resume flow at prescribed rate.

17. If the additive has an oil–lipid base, mix the admixture every 15 to 20 minutes during the infusion by gentle rotation of the container.

18. If adding medication to a vented glass infusate container that is already hung, it is essential to disconnect the air vent from the primary tubing, insert the syringe into the air vent port, inject medication into the bottle, replace the air vent, and gently rotate the bottle to ensure mixing. Maintain strict aseptic technique throughout manipulation.

19. Use a long needle when injecting a drug into a port on the administration set to minimize the amount of drug that is trapped in the port.

20. Maintain IV tubing in a position that is level with or above the patient's IV site to prevent backflow of drug through the tubing.

Antibiotics: Nursing Implications

General Nursing Interventions

1. Review the literature to ensure that the antibiotic ordered and method of administration are consistent with the patient's infection.

2. Check the package expiration date.

3. Review reconstitution, dilution, and storage information.

4. Correctly label the admixture by including drug name, concentration, diluent, date, time, and initials.

5. Ensure familiarity with the potential adverse effects of the drug.

6. Review the patient's allergies.

7. Use strict aseptic techniques throughout administration.

8. Administer the drug at the specified times to ensure maintenance of the proper drug level.

9. Thoroughly assess/monitor functions of the organ(s) that metabolize the antibiotic.
10. Always evaluate the patient for sensitivity to the drug.
11. Be prepared to respond to anaphylaxis, which can occur from within a few seconds of administration to 30 minutes following administration.
12. Signs and symptoms of anaphylaxis are the following:
    - Diffuse flushing
    - Itching
    - Feeling of warmth
    - Hives
    - Respiratory difficulty
    - Abdominal cramping
    - Urinary/bowel incontinence
    - Possible respiratory/circulatory failure
13. Use the following nursing interventions for anaphylaxis:
    - Immediately stop the infusion.
    - Establish the airway.
    - Notify the physician.
    - Apply a tourniquet above the injection site and administer epinephrine.
    - Administer drugs as ordered to include antihistamines, vasopressors, and others.
14. Review Table 14-1 for selected antibiotics and related nursing interventions.

Antineoplastic Agents: Nursing Implications

Definition of Chemotherapy

Toxic, antineoplastic agents are administered for the purpose of destroying malignant cells through their specific or nonspecific effect on the cell life cycle. Chemotherapy can be given in an attempt to cure the patient, control the spread of disease, or postpone recurrence of disease.

Table 14-1. Selected Antibiotics and Related Nursing Interventions

Antibiotic Category	Selected Nursing Interventions
Aminoglycosides	Assess for muscle weakness
	Closely monitor renal function
	Carefully assess balance and hearing functions
	Note that IV route can cause excessive blood levels
Cephalosporins	Exercise caution if more than one is used concurrently because of additive nephrotoxic effects
	Do not administer if patient has history of penicillin sensitivity
	Rotate sites often, since phlebitis is common following administration
	Closely monitor renal function
Chloramphenicol	Only administer intravenously
	Assess for risk of irreversible aplastic anemia
	Closely monitor bone marrow function
Clindamycin/ Lincomycin	Monitor hepatic function
	Use precautions to prevent phlebitis
Erythromycin	Use precautions to prevent phlebitis
	This antibiotic is among the safest of all antibiotics
Penicillins	Implement precautions for phlebitis
	Monitor neurologic status when administering penicillin G
	Never administer procaine penicillin by IV route
Spectinomycin	Monitor hemoglobin/hematocrit values
	Monitor renal function
Tetracyclines	Do not administer to patient with history of liver disorders

Continued

Table 14-1. (Continued)

Antibiotic Category	Selected Nursing Interventions
	Generally contraindicated for patients with renal failure
	Assess for development of superinfections
Vancomycin	Implement precautions for phlebitis
	Monitor renal function
	Monitor auditory function
	Administer dosage (500 mg) over at least 60 minutes because of the potential severity of reactions
	Monitor blood pressure during infusion
Amphotericin B	Closely monitor for signs of thrombophlebitis
	Monitor renal function
	Reconstitute with sterile water *without* preservatives or bacteriostatic agents
	Note that this drug is incompatible with most other medications
	Avoid most in-line filters since the large drug particles may become trapped in the filter
	Cover bottle with paper bag or wrap with foil since drug deteriorates rapidly when exposed to direct/indirect sunlight
	Use strict aseptic techniques

Life Cycle of the Cell

The life cycle of the cell consists of the following five phases:

1. G_0. Cells perform their designated activity but are at rest.
2. G_1. Cells begin the process of reproduction; possible production of ribonucleic acid (RNA) occurs.

3. S. Cells continue the process in preparation for re-production by synthesizing deoxyribonucleic acid (DNA). This phase lasts 6 to 8 hours.
4. G_2. Cells receive additional synthesized RNA.
5. M. Cells divide and reproduce.

Classification of Antineoplastic Drugs

1. Antineoplastic agents can be classified into groups according to common characteristics. Table 14-2 summarizes these groups.
2. The cell-cycle-specific and cell-cycle-nonspecific classifications are one way of categorizing anticancer drugs. Cell-cycle-specific drugs refer to the antineo-plastic drugs that can destroy only actively dividing cells. It excludes those agents that are effective dur-ing the G_0 phase. Drug groupings that are cell-cycle specific include
   · Antimetabolites
   · Plant alkaloids
3. Cell-cycle-nonspecific drugs include those agents that can destroy cells in all 5 phases. Drug groupings that are cell-cycle nonspecific include
   · Alkylating agents
   · Antitumor antibiotics
   · Steroids
   · Nitrosureas

Patient Eligibility Criteria for Chemotherapy

· Tumor susceptibility
· State of disease
· Patient's clinical status
· Potential for quality of life

General Guidelines for Administration of IV Antineoplastic Agents (Hughes, 1986)

1. Acquire advanced knowledge and skill in administra-tion of antineoplastic agents.
2. Establish a therapeutic, caring relationship.

Table 14-2. Classification of Antineoplastic Drugs

Classification	Definition	Common Drugs
Alkylating agents	Interfere with DNA synthesis throughout the cell life cycle	Mechlorethamine (Mustargen)
		Cyclophosphamide (Cytoxan)
		Triethylenethiophosphoramide (TSPA, Thiotepa)
Antimetabolites	Work within the cell cycle in the S phase	Fluorouracil (5-FU)
		Methotrexate (Mexate)
		Cytarabine (Cytosar-U)
		Etoposide (VePesid)
Antibiotics	Thought to inhibit DNA or RNA synthesis	Doxorubicin HCL (Adriamycin)
		Bleomycin (Blenoxane)
		Mithramycin (Mithracin)
		Mitomycin-C (Mutamycin)
		Dactinomycin (actinomycin D, Cosmegen)
Steroids	Thought to alter the cell environment because of their chemical semblance to hormonal agents	Diethylstilbestrol (Stilphostrol)
		Celestone phosphate (Betamethasone)
Plant alkaloids	Act during the M phase by preventing mitosis	Vinblastine (Velban)
		Vincristine (Oncovin)
Nitrosureas	Highly lipid soluble, can cross blood–brain barrier	Dacarbazine (DTIC-Dome)
		Cisplatin (Platinol)
		Carmustine (BCNU)

- · Use therapeutic verbal and nonverbal communication skills.
- · Maintain eye contact.
- · Involve friends, relatives, and significant others in care.
- · Support spiritual needs.
3. Complete a thorough patient health assessment prior to initiating therapy.
4. Ensure that a signed consent form for administering investigational agents is present on the chart.
5. Initiate a teaching plan that includes the following:
    - · Information related to resources of the American Cancer Society, National Cancer Institute
    - · Drug information including purpose, administration, and complications of the agents.
    - · Consideration of the disease process, patient's ability to comprehend instructions, family setting, and cooperation of the patient's physician (Hedrick, 1984).
6. Review the physician's order. The RN administering medication should check drug, dosage, and route with another RN; both RNs should go to the patient to verify correct identification.
7. Prepare all chemotherapy drugs under a laminar flow hood to provide for air venting.
8. Use disposable, closed-front, moisture-barrier gowns with elastic or knit cuffs, latex gloves (change every 30 minutes), masks, and safety glasses or eyeglasses.
9. Adhere to strict aseptic technique throughout preparation and administration.
10. Control drippage and production of aerosol.
    - · Use the laminar flow hood.
    - · Clear fluid or powder from top portion of the container.
    - · Use a syringe large enough that following drawing up of the drug the syringe is no more than three-fourths full.
    - · Open containers in a direction away from self.

- Always hold the bevel of the needle away from self.
- Do not inject air into the vial prior to withdrawing the drug.
- After withdrawing the drug with the syringe, allow air to flow back into the vial before withdrawing the needle from the vial.
- Always maintain negative pressure within the vial to prevent spraying of the drug.
- Do not expel excess air while holding the syringe at eye level.
- Place an alcohol swab at the needle tip while expelling excess air.

11. Put on sterile gloves.
12. Ensure a patent IV infusion site by instilling 1 ml to 2 ml saline. It is preferable to use a new IV site for each administration, since repeated use may lead to drug leakage or loss of patency.
13. Use the smallest-gauge needles (23–25), if not contraindicated, for administration.
14. Ascertain patency throughout administration.
15. Use a saline flush following administration to avoid drug admixture problems and leakage of drug from the needle/port.
16. Following administration, remove the needle and apply pressure with a sterile 2 × 2-inch gauze for 3 to 4 minutes.
17. Observe meticulously for extravasation.
18. Be prepared to respond to severe allergic reactions that may accompany certain agents.
19. Consider any used/unused chemotherapy drug products/containers and related gloves/masks as toxic chemical waste and dispose of according to Environmental Protection Agency recommendations.
20. Document in the chart the medication, dosage, and site where administered, as well as the patient's reactions.

Selected Complications of Chemotherapy

1. Phlebitis (see Chapter 8)
2. Vein flare
   - A localized allergic reaction to doxorubicin (Adriamycin) (Troutman, 1985)
   - Weltlike patches, itching, burning along vein
3. Extravasation
   - Most dangerous complication
   - Leakage of drug solution into area around injection site resulting in necrosis of soft tissue, nerves, blood vessels
   - Signs and symptoms include the following:
     Pain
     Swelling
     Inflammation
     Burning
     Erythema
     Soreness at site
     Induration, thrombophlebitis, venous discoloration
     Necrosis
   - The most damaging antineoplastic drugs are the vesicants, agents that cause sloughing and necrosis. Common vesicants and related antidotes are summarized in Table 14-3 (Faehnrich, 1984; Wetmore, 1985). See specific institutional policies for administration procedures.
   - Nursing interventions for extravasation are the following:
     Stop the IV infusion.
     Leave the needle in place.
     Withdraw 4 ml to 5 ml of blood.
     Administer the specific antidote, if indicated (see Table 14-3).
     Inject lidocaine/local anesthetic according to institutional policy, if indicated.
     Remove the IV line. Pack the site in ice for 15 to

Table 14-3. Common Vesicants and Related Antidotes

Vesicant	Antidote
Actinomycin (dactinomycin, Cosmegen)	Sodium thiosulfate, 10%—4 ml Ascorbic acid, 50 mg/ml—5 ml
Carmustine (BCNU)	Sodium bicarbonate, 8.4%—5 ml
Daunorubicin (Cerubidine, daunomycin)	Sodium bicarbonate, 8.4%—5 ml Dexamethasone, 4 mg/ml—1 ml
Mitomycin (Mutamycin)	Sodium thiosulfate, 10%—4 ml Ascorbic acid, 50 mg/ml—1 ml
Mithramycin (Mithracin)	Edetate disodium 150 mg/ml—1 ml
Nitrogen mustard (Mustargen)	Sodium thiosulfate, 10%—4 ml
Vinblastine (Velban)	Hyaluronidase, 150 units/ml—4 ml Sodium bicarbonate, or 4%—5 ml
Vincristine (Oncovin)	Hyaluronidase, 150 units/ml—1 ml Sodium bicarbonate, 8.4%—5 ml

20 minutes every 4 to 6 hours, for up to 72 hours; or apply cold compresses to the area every hour for 24 hours to reduce inflammation and localize tissue destruction as ordered by physician (Dozier and Ballentine, 1983; Nurse Drug Alert, 1985; Stephens, 1983).

Note: It is suggested that hot compresses be used with vincristine, vinblastine, or mithramycin, since the heat will disperse the enzymatic drug activity in the tissues and allow for increased blood flow to move the drug away from the local area (Faehnrich, 1984).

- Nursing interventions to prevent extravasation are the following:

Limit performance of venipuncture to experienced personnel only.

Use new IV sites for each administration, if possible.

Avoid IV sites near joints, lower extremities, areas of previous radiation therapy.

Maintain visibility of site.

Ensure patency before administration.

Aspirate frequently.

Administer the appropriate dilution over the shortest time consistent with the patient's venous capacity.

Meticulously monitor the infusion.

Observe the IV site carefully.

Assess patient response.

Use saline flush following administration.

If administering more than one agent, administer the nonvesicant first; follow each drug with 3 ml to 5 ml of normal saline fluid.

4. One or more of the following complications may result from specific antineoplastic drugs:

- Diarrhea
- Fever
- Gastrointestinal bleeding/ulceration
- Leukopenia
- Nausea/vomiting
- Neurologic changes
- Stomatitis
- Thrombocytopenia
- Thromboembolism
- Low therapeutic index
- Complications related to rapidly proliferating tissues
- Organ toxicities
- Psychosocial complications

Continuous Narcotic Infusions (CNI)

1. Purpose includes the following:
   - Control of pain
   - Possibly patient control
2. Advantages include the following:
   - Extending control of rate of administration to the patient to accommodate individual variations
   - Almost immediate relief
3. Medications used include the following:
   - Morphine (less expensive) (Dolby and White-stone, 1985)
   - Leoorphanol tartrate (Levo-Dromoran)
   - Methadone
4. Nursing interventions are as follows:
   - Select the client carefully.
   - Use the infusion pump or volume control set.
   - Initiate infusion of 25 ml of infusate with 1-hour dose of the drug and run at 25 ml/hr.
   - Repeat the above for the second hour.
   - If the client is comfortable, place on a 4-hour schedule by using 100 ml of infusate and a 4-hour dose of the drug.
   - Assess the client at least every 30 minutes, especially noting comfort level and respiratory status.
   - If respiratory rate falls below 14/min, decrease the IV by 50% and notify the physician (O'Donnell and Papciak, 1981).
   - Document through the use of a flow sheet.

Refer to the Bibliography for additional information related to the administration of critical-care medications.

Bibliography

Adams S: Alternative chemotherapeutic administration. Infusion 7:115–122, 1983

Baaske I, Amann A, Wagenknecht D et al: Nitroglycerin compatibility with intravenous fluid filter containers and administration sets. Am J Hosp Pharm 37(2):201, 1980

Bergemann D: Handling antineoplastic agents. Am J Intravenous Ther Clin Nutr 16:13–17, 1983

Bledsoe L: Antineoplastic agents—management of health risks for the I.V. nurse. NITA 6(5):332, 1983

Carlson K: IV antibiotics. NITA 9:62, January/February 1986

Coblio N: Don't combine those drugs! Nursing81, 11:48–49, 1981

Cohen M: Stay with the patient after giving the first dose of an I.V. drug. Nursing86, 16:23, 1986

Comer J: Amphotericin B: Ten common questions. Am J Nurs 11:1166–1167, 1981

Conway G: Intravenous piggyback admixture: Guidelines for infusion and stability. Infusion 10(2):28, 1986

Dolby B, Whitestone S: Continuous morphine drip for intractable pain control. NITA 8(5):415, 1985

Dozier N, Ballentine R: Practical considerations in the preparation and administration of cancer chemotherapy. Am Intravenous Ther Clin Nutr 16:6–31, 1983

Drew D, Schumann D: Homogeneity of potassium chloride in small volume intravenous containers. Nurs Res 35(6):325, 1986

Embury S, Davison L, Miller R: Using a microcomputer for intravenous drug protocols. Appl Pharmacol 4(4): 226, 1985

Faehnrich J: Extravasation. NITA 7(1):49, 1984

Hans P, Paris P, Mathot R: Intravenous nitroglycerin perfusion techniques—clinical implications. Intensive Care Med 8(2):93, 1982

Hedrick C: Patient teaching: Side effects of chemotherapy. NITA 7(3):178, 1984

Hughes C: Giving cancer drugs IV: Some guidelines. Am J Nurs 86:34–38, 1986

Jameson J, O'Donnell J: Guidelines for extravasation of intravenous drugs. Infusion 7(5):157, 1983

Johnston S, Patt Y: Intraarterial chemotherapy. Nursing81, 11:108–112, 1981

Koza C: Principles and practices of cancer chemotherapy. NITA 6:326, September/October 1983

Langslet J, Habel M: The aminoglycoside antibiotics. Am J Nurs, pp 1144–1146, June 1981

Leff R: Intravenous administration of medications to the pediatric patient. NITA 6:255, July/August 1983

Levitt D: Cancer chemotherapy. RN 44:69–72, 1981

Lira C: Nursing implications of anti-neoplastic drugs. Infusion 8:15, January/February 1984

McCollam P, Garrison T: Etoposide: A new chemotherapeutic agent. Am J Intravenous Ther Clin Nutr 17:24–28, March 1984

McGuire L, Wright A: Continuous narcotic infusion. Nursing84, 14:50–55, December 1984

Mark L: The "puff technique" for intravenous diazepam. Anesthesiology 61:630, 1984

Markowitz J, Pearson G, Kay B et al: Nurses, physicians, and pharmacists: Their knowledge of hazards of medication. Nurs Res 30(6):366, 1981

Miller B, Peska L: The effect of freezing on particulate matter concentrations in five antibiotic solutions. Am J Intravenous Ther Clin Nutr 17:19–22, 1984

Moore R, Terry B: Nafcillin necrosis. NITA 7(1):61, 1984

Morris M: Intravenous drug incompatibilities. Am J Nurs 79:1288, 1979

Motz-Harding E, Good F: The right solution—mixing IV drugs thoroughly. Nursing85 15:62–64, 1985

Newton M, Gilbert J, Newton D: Parenteral antibiotics. RN 44:45–51, 1981

Nurse Drug Alert: Managing extravasation wounds caused by antineoplastic drugs. NITA Update 6(6):6, 1985

O'Donnell J: An introduction to adverse drug reactions. Infusion 9(4):112, 1985

O'Donnell L, Papciak B: Continuous morphine infusion for controlling intractable pain. Nursing81, 11:69–12, 1981

Raymond G, Day P: Administration set purging for dosage adjustments in intravenous nitroglycerin therapy. NITA 6(6):415, 1983

Sesin P, Wiggins M: New England Deaconess guidelines for the administration of I.V. drugs. NITA 10(1):17, 1987

Seymour F: Parenteral chemotherapeutic agents. NITA 8:207, May/June 1985

Silverman H: Narcotic analgesic drugs and patient controlled analgesia. Special Delivery 2(2):1, 1986

Simone P, Linkewich J: Guidelines for administration of parenteral drugs. Am J IV Ther Clin Nutr 8:19–24, 1981

Smith B: Patient-controlled analgesia: Its uses and benefits. Intravenous Ther News 12(9):7, 1985

Stephens B: Kennestone Hospital policies and guidelines for preparing and administering cytotoxic drugs. NITA 6:433, November/December 1983

Terry J: Syringe pump delivery bolus meds. NITA Update 7(2):5, 1986

Trester A, Nader M: Guide for the administration and use of cancer chemotherapeutic agents. Am J IV Ther Clin Nutr 9:9–31, 1982.

Trissel L: Evaluation of the literature on stability and compatibility of parenteral admixtures. NITA 8(4):365, 1985

Troutman J: Step-by-step guide to trouble-free IV chemotherapy. RN 48:32–34, 1985

Tschampel M, Clouse J, Visconti J: Intravenous push medications which qualified registered nurses may administer. Intravenous Ther News, p 3, August 1984

Turco S: Adsorption of insulin in infusion containers and tubing. Am J Intravenous Ther Clin Nutr 9:44–48, 1982

Turco S, Rock M: The effects of microwave radiation on frozen parenteral antibiotics: A review. Parenterals 2:1–6, 1984

Valanis B, Browne M: Use of protection by nurses during occupational handling of antineoplastic drugs. NITA 8(3):218, 1985

Valenzano L: Utilization of a standard form for the administration of cis-platinum in a community hospital. NITA 7(6):515, 1984

Vohra S, Aggarwal P, O'Donnell J: Guidelines for compatibility of IV additives. Infusion 8:8, 1984

Wagner W: Current concepts of I.V. nitroglycerin therapy. NITA 6(5):342, 1983

Wetmore N: 1985. Extravasation—the dreaded complication. NITA 8(1):47, 1985

Wisniewski B: The three C's of administering chemotherapy. NITA 9:22, January/February 1986

15 ▷ Administration of Blood and Blood Products

Key Points

1. Basic immunohematology
2. Blood products available
3. Administration procedures for blood and blood products
4. Complications

Basic Immunohematology

Transfusion therapy consists in the introduction of whole blood or blood products directly into the circulation of a patient for therapeutic purposes, which may include the following:

1. To improve the oxygen-carrying capacity of the blood
2. To restore circulating blood volume following injury or burns
3. To replace specific clotting factors or cellular components
4. To treat shock

Blood Grouping Systems

Human blood can be typed on the basis of the presence or absence of certain antigens and antibodies. Several different blood grouping systems are used to type blood.

1. ABO system
   - This is the most important system in transfusion therapy.

- Human blood groups are inherited; groups are determined by which antigens are present on the surfaces of red blood cells (RBCs) and which antibodies are present in the plasma.
- A patient who needs blood must first have a blood group determination done to identify which antigens and antibodies are present in his blood.
- Once the patient's blood type has been identified, a unit of donor blood of the proper compatible type can be selected.
- The following chart summarizes blood group determination and donor–recipient compatibility:

Blood Type	Recipient Antigens Present on RBCs	Antibodies Present in Plasma	Compatible Donor Type
A	A	Anti-B	A, O
B	B	Anti-A	B, O
AB	A and B	None	A, B, AB, and O
O	None	Anti-A and anti-B	O

2. Rh system
   - This is the second most important system in transfusion therapy.
   - Rh antigens are also inherited and found on the surface of RBCs.
   - The strongest and most important Rh antigen is the D antigen.
   - 85% of the population have the D antigen; these persons are called Rh positive; persons lacking the D antigen are called Rh negative.
   - Rh-positive persons lack anti-D antibodies.
   - Rh-negative persons also lack anti-D antibodies, but if an Rh-negative person becomes immunized against the D antigen through transfusion with Rh-positive blood or through pregnancy, the Rh-negative person will develop antibodies against the D antigen.

- If the immunized Rh-negative person receives a subsequent transfusion with Rh-positive blood, a transfusion reaction could occur, or if an Rh-negative woman delivers an Rh-positive infant, and if during delivery RBCs from the infant (these cells will carry the D antigen that the mother's RBCs lack) enter the mother's circulation, she will make anti-D antibodies; although this infant will be unaffected, subsequent Rh-positive infants may be affected with hemolytic disease of the newborn (HDN).
- In both of these cases, the Rh-negative person receiving Rh-positive blood and the Rh-negative woman giving birth to an Rh-positive infant, production of anti-D antibodies could be stopped by the administration of Rh immune globulin (RhIG); this globulin coats the D antigen and blocks the formation of anti-D antibodies.

3. HLA (human leukocyte antigen) system
   - This system is very complex and is used mainly in matching tissues for transplantation.
   - HLA is located on the surface of circulating white blood cells, platelets, and most tissue cells.
   - HLA typing is sometimes done to identify and select donors of platelets and granulocytes for patients who have received multiple units of either of these components and have become immunized against those tissue antigens.
   - Since HLA is inherited, it can be used in paternity testing.

Blood Products Available

Whole Blood

Description and Shelf Life
1. Each 500-ml unit consists of approximately 200 ml of RBCs and approximately 300 ml of plasma.
2. The unit can be stored for 21, 35, or 42 days (depending on the anticoagulant-preservative solution used) at 4°C.

Indications for Use
1. Massive transfusion following acute blood loss (usually blood loss of a liter or more)
2. Neonatal exchange transfusion

Equipment Recommendations
1. Blood administration set with in-line blood filter of standard size (pore size 170 μ); for some patients (neonates, patients with compromised pulmonary status, multiple-unit recipients) microaggregate filters (pore size 20μ–40μ) should be used
2. Multiple-lead tubing (Y set is best) with normal saline (0.9% sodium chloride) for starter solution
3. Large-gauge needle or plastic catheter (18- or 19-gauge for most adults and 21-, 22-, or 23-gauge for infants and children, geriatric patients, or adults who are dehydrated or undergoing long-term IV therapy, chemotherapy, or radiation therapy)

Administration Techniques
1. Obtain the blood product no more than 30 minutes before the expected time of administration; caution staff members who transport the product that crushing or manipulating the blood bag can damage the cells.
2. Follow established procedures *to the letter* for identifying blood product and patient (usually two or more persons must do this).
3. Take the patient's baseline vital signs.
4. Always use *strict aseptic technique* in performing transfusion.
5. Put on sterile gloves.
6. Start the transfusion *slowly* at a rate of about 2 ml/min, and give no more than 30 ml during the first 15 minutes.
7. Observe the patient carefully for any signs or symptoms of discomfort or adverse reaction (Tables 15-1 and 15-2).
8. Administer absolutely *no* medications or drugs along with the blood product.

9. If no problems occur during the first 15 minutes, adjust the rate of administration to what was prescribed; the complete unit should be given within 2 to 4 hours.
10. Gently agitate the blood product during administration.
11. Continue to monitor the patient's vital signs throughout the transfusion.

Special Nursing Interventions

1. Always administer ABO-group-specific and Rh-type-specific whole blood.
2. A single unit of whole blood has questionable therapeutic value—component or derivative therapy may be more appropriate.
3. If the physician ordered whole blood but the laboratory tends to send packed RBCs, ask the physician to specify which is preferred.
4. AIDS (acquired immunodeficiency syndrome)
   • Since early 1983, blood donors considered to be members of a high-risk group for AIDS have been asked not to donate blood (Zuck, 1986); these high-risk groups include the following (Jaffe, 1986):
   Homosexual or bisexual men
   IV drug users
   Patients with hemophilia or other coagulation disorders
   Patients who have received transfusions
   Heterosexuals whose sexual partners include members of the above groups
   • Since the spring of 1985, all donated blood and plasma units have been screened with an enzyme immunoassay (EIA) for the presence of antibodies to the AIDS virus (this virus is known by several names: HTLV-III/LAV [human T-cell lymphotropic virus type III/lymphadenopathy-associated virus] and HIV [human immunodeficiency virus] are two that are frequently used) (Curran et al, 1985);

any blood unit found positive for the AIDS virus is discarded and not transfused or used to make any other blood component or product.

- Because of these precautions, the blood supply is considered to be very safe (Zuck, 1986), but since the incubation period of AIDS can be as long as 5 years, a small number of AIDS cases in hemophiliacs and recipients of blood transfusions may continue to be reported in those who have already become infected since the time that these precautions were begun (Curran et al, 1985).
- At this time, no treatment, vaccine, or cure for AIDS is known (Public Health Service, 1986); therefore, strict adherence to donor screening procedures, voluntary donor exclusion, and EIA screening of donated units must be maintained to decrease the risk of transmission of the AIDS virus by transfusion.
- See the Bibliography for further information about AIDS.

Packed Red Blood Cells

Description and Shelf Life

1. Each 250-ml unit consists of approximately 200 ml of RBCs and 50 ml of plasma.
2. The hematocrit of a unit of packed RBCs ranges from 70% to 85%.
3. Each unit of packed RBCs can be expected to raise the average nonbleeding adult patient's hematocrit 3% and the hemoglobin 1g/dl.
4. The shelf life is the same as for whole blood, but if the unit is opened it must be used within 24 hours.

Indications for Use

1. To restore or increase the oxygen-carrying capacity of blood and to increase red cell mass
2. To treat acute anemia, aplastic anemia, and some chronic anemias

Equipment Recommendations

1. Recommendations are the same as for whole blood, but since packed RBCs are more viscous than whole blood, a filter with a larger surface area may be used to increase the transfusion rate.

2. If there is a physician's order, 50 ml of normal saline may be added to the unit aseptically thru a Y set to decrease its viscosity. This should be done *only* if the patient is in no danger of fluid overload; the additional fluid should be recorded in the patient's chart.

Administration Techniques

1. Administration is the same as for whole blood.

2. The product should be gently agitated more frequently during administration to help maintain the infusion rate.

Special Nursing Interventions

1. Always administer ABO-group-specific and Rh-type-specific product; if this is not available, ABO-group- and Rh-type-compatible product may usually be given.

2. See Special Nursing Interventions in the section on whole blood for notes on AIDS.

Leukocyte-Poor Red Blood Cells

Leukocyte-poor RBCs include cells prepared by inverted centrifugation, washing, and freezing/deglycerolizing.

Description and Shelf Life

1. Leukocyte-poor RBCs can be prepared by the inverted centrifugation technique; units prepared this way have 70% of all leukocytes and platelets removed, but there is also a loss of 20% of the red cells; if prepared in a closed system, the unit retains the same expiration time and storage requirements as packed RBCs.

2. Washed RBCs contain very few leukocytes, platelets, or microaggregates and very little plasma; a 250-ml unit is stored at 4°C and must be used within 24 hours after washing.
3. Frozen deglycerolized RBCs have lower levels of leukocytes, platelets, and microaggregates than any other leukocyte-poor red cell component and contain virtually no plasma; a 250-ml unit can be stored frozen for 3 years; a thawed unit is stored at 4°C and must be used within 24 hours after thawing.

Indications for Use
1. For patients who have developed HLA antibodies to leukocytes, for multiparous women, for patients needing multiple transfusions, and for transfusion during transplant surgery
2. Washed RBCs for prevention of febrile nonhemolytic transfusion reactions due to leukocyte antibodies; IgA (immunoglobulin A) deficiency with sensitivity to IgA
3. Frozen deglycerolized RBCs used same as washed RBCs; also to supply rare blood types and as storage method for autologous transfusion

Equipment Recommendations
1. Recommendations are the same as for whole blood.
2. A microaggregate filter is usually not indicated, since most plasma constituents and microaggregates are eliminated by the washing procedures.

Administration Techniques
1. Administration is the same as for whole blood.

Special Nursing Interventions
1. Always administer ABO-group-specific and Rh-type-specific product; if this is unavailable, ABO-group- and Rh-type-compatible product may be given.
2. Since very little plasma and very few leukocytes are infused with these RBCs, there is reduced risk of

HLA and protein sensitization and fewer febrile, anaphylactic, and allergic reactions.
3. Leukocyte-poor red cell preparations are usually very expensive to prepare.
4. See Special Nursing Interventions in the section on whole blood for notes on AIDS.

Platelet Concentrate

Description and Shelf Life

1. A 30-ml to 50-ml unit of random donor platelet concentrate contains approximately 5.5×10^{10} platelets suspended in approximately 50 ml of plasma and can be expected to raise the platelet count approximately 9,000 to 10,000/μl in a 70-kg adult; platelet concentrates can be stored at room temperature (20°C to 24°C) under continuous gentle agitation for 3 to 5 days, depending on the type of storage container.
2. A 350-ml unit containing approximately 3 to 8×10^{11} platelets in approximately 300 ml of plasma can be expected to raise the platelet count by 50,000 to 100,000/μl in a 70-kg adult patient and can be harvested from a single donor using the technique of plateletpheresis; since collection by this method does not take place in a closed system, these platelets must be used within 24 hours.

Indications for Use

1. For treatment of nondestructive thrombocytopenia, platelet dysfunction, aplastic anemia, bone marrow depression, and bleeding in thrombocytopenic patients
2. Also indicated when massive hemorrhage has caused thrombocytopenia owing to rapid dilution of platelets following administration of whole blood or resuscitation fluids

Equipment Recommendations

1. Recommendations are the same as for whole blood, except microaggregate filters cannot be used because they tend to trap platelets.

2. Special platelet administration sets (component syringe and component drip) are available that contain a smaller filter and shorter rubber-free tubing to minimize platelet attraction; Y-type sets will allow the platelet pack to be flushed with normal saline for maximum platelet infusion.
3. Use of an 18- or 19-gauge needle is recommended for rapid infusion.

Administration Techniques
1. Administration is the same as for whole blood, but platelets should be given more rapidly, at a rate of approximately 5 to 10 minutes per concentrate.
2. The platelet bag must be gently agitated repeatedly during administration to minimize platelet clumping.

Special Nursing Interventions
1. Administer ABO-group- and Rh-type-compatible concentrate when possible; if this is not available, unmatched platelets may be given.
2. Patients on long-term platelet therapy who have become immunized may need HLA typing.
3. Monitor the patient for possible allergic or febrile reactions during transfusion, although these will usually be minor.
4. See Special Nursing Interventions in the section on whole blood for notes on AIDS.

Granulocytes

Description and Shelf Life
1. Approximately 10^{10} granulocytes can be collected from a single donor by leukapheresis techniques into units of varying size from 200 ml to 500 ml; the majority of cells collected are granulocytes, but lymphocytes, monocytes, platelets, and RBCs will also be present in small numbers.
2. Granulocytes should be given immediately but can be held up to 24 hours without agitation at 20°C to 24°C.

Indications for Use
1. For granulocytopenic patients with progressive infections that are not responsive to antibiotics; agranulocytic patients with gram-negative bacteremia or progressive infection; oncology patients with severe bone marrow depression
2. Prophylactic granulocytic transfusion is currently controversial.

Equipment Recommendations
1. Recommendations are the same as for whole blood, except the use of a microaggregate filter is contraindicated because it can trap granulocytes.

Administration Techniques
1. Administration is the same as for whole blood, except granulocytes should be given at a slower rate of 1 unit over 2 to 4 hours to minimize transfusion reactions.

Special Nursing Interventions
1. Administer ABO-group- and Rh-type-compatible product when possible; some clients may require HLA typing if they have become sensitized from previous transfusions.
2. Granulocytes must be administered daily for 4 to 7 days or more to be effective; a one-time dose of a single unit has questionable therapeutic value.
3. Be alert for reactions that frequently occur in clients receiving granulocytes, such as fever, chills, or hives; these reactions can usually be treated symptomatically with acetaminophen or an antihistamine and are not cause for transfusion termination.
4. If severe hypotension, anaphylactic response, or severe respiratory reaction similar to pulmonary embolism should occur, stop the transfusion immediately, keep a vein open, and notify the physician.
5. See Special Nursing Interventions in the section on whole blood for notes on AIDS.

Fresh Frozen Plasma (FFP)

Description and Shelf Life

1. A 200-ml to 250-ml unit of plasma containing all coagulation factors (but no platelets) is separated from a unit of whole blood within 6 hours of collection and frozen rapidly to maintain stability of labile coagulation factors.
2. FFP can be stored at $-18°C$ for 12 months; once thawed, it must be used within 2 hours or coagulation factors can deteriorate.

Indications for Use

1. Plasma volume expansion
2. Treatment of inherited or acquired coagulation disorders, hypovolemic shock, bleeding complications due to liver disease

Equipment Recommendations

1. Recommendations are the same as for whole blood, but a microaggregate filter is contraindicated because it could trap plasma.
2. Use of a component administration set that contains a smaller-surface-area filter may decrease plasma trapping.
3. A smaller-gauge needle may be used.

Administration Techniques

1. Administration is the same as for whole blood, but the unit must be given within 2 hours after thawing.

Special Nursing Interventions

1. Always administer ABO-group-specific or ABO-group-compatible product. (Rh type compatibility is unnecessary since FFP contains no RBCs.)
2. Monitor the patient for possible febrile or allergic reactions.
3. Remember that a unit of FFP requires 20 minutes to thaw before it can be administered.

4. FFP carries the same risk of hepatitis transmission as a unit of blood and should not be given when simple crystalloid therapy would be adequate.
5. See Special Nursing Interventions in the section on whole blood for notes on AIDS.

Cryoprecipitate

Description and Shelf Life
1. A 10-ml to 20-ml cryoprecipitate is prepared by thawing FFP under refrigeration and physically removing the cryoprecipitate.
2. A single-donor cryoprecipitate contains at least 80 International Units (IU) of Factor VIII and approximately 250 mg of fibrinogen in approximately 10 ml to 15 ml of plasma.
3. Cryoprecipitate can be stored for 1 year at $-18°C$; once thawed it should be given as soon as possible but can be held for 6 hours at $22°C$.

Indications for Use
1. Hemophilia A
2. von Willebrand's disease
3. Fibrinogen replacement
4. Control of bleeding associated with Factor VIII deficiency

Equipment Recommendations
1. Recommendations are the same as for whole blood, except the use of a component Y set is recommended so that normal saline can be used to flush the pack after transfusion.
2. A smaller-gauge needle may be used.

Administration Techniques
1. Administration is the same as for whole blood, except cryoprecipitate should be infused more rapidly (usually at a rate of one 10-ml–20-ml cryoprecipitate in 5 minutes) to prevent deterioration of coagulation factors.

2. Treatment usually consists of several cryoprecipitates given per dose (based on patient's weight), with two to three doses given each day for several days.

Special Nursing Interventions

1. Administer ABO-group-compatible product when possible. (Rh type compatibility is unnecessary.)
2. Complications include an increased risk of hepatitis (1 cryoprecipitate carries the same hepatitis risk as 1 unit of blood, but since multiple cryoprecipitates are given together, the risk is increased), occasional urticarial reactions, and occasional vasomotor reactions (a type of febrile reaction that produces chills, slight fever, and headache; generally more uncomfortable than dangerous and medication usually not administered).
3. See Special Nursing Interventions in the section on whole blood for notes on AIDS.
4. Antibodies to the AIDS virus have been detected in hemophiliac patients treated with cryoprecipitate (Gjerset et al, 1985; Gjerset et al, 1984; Levy et al, 1984); careful screening of all donated blood products should help decrease the risk of AIDS transmission.
5. The National Hemophilia Foundation Medical and Scientific Advisory Council, in their *Medical Bulletin #15,* October 13, 1984, listed recommendations for the prevention of AIDS in hemophiliacs, including the use of heat-treated factor concentrates that have had the AIDS virus inactivated during the manufacturing process (Rutman and Miller, 1985).

Factor VIII Concentrate and Factor IX Concentrate

Description and Shelf Life

1. Factor VIII concentrate is a commercially available lyophilized plasma derivative that contains only Factor VIII. It is available in different concentrations based on the number of Factor VIII International Units per vial, up to 1000 units. In the lyophilized form it can be stored for 2 years at 2°C to 8°C; once

reconstituted, it should be administered within 3 hours.

2. Factor IX concentrate (also known as prothrombin complex concentrate) is a commercially available lyophilized plasma derivative that contains high levels of the vitamin K–dependent factors (Factors II [prothrombin], VII, IX, and X); the concentration of Factor IX usually ranges from 400 IU to 500 IU per vial and is reconstituted with 10 ml to 20 ml of diluent. In the lyophilized form it can be stored for 2 years at 2°C to 8°C; once reconstituted, it should be given within 3 hours.

Indications for Use

1. Factor VIII concentrate is used to treat hemophilia A.
2. Factor IX concentrate is used to treat hemophilia B.

Equipment Recommendations

1. Recommendations are the same as for whole blood, except a component syringe set and smaller-gauge needle may be used.

Administration Techniques

1. Administration is the same as for whole blood, except factor concentrates can be administered at a faster rate.
2. Usually only one person is needed for identification of product and patient.

Special Nursing Interventions

1. ABO group and Rh type compatibility are unnecessary.
2. Complications include a very high risk of hepatitis transmission with both concentrates; the incidence of vasomotor reactions following transfusion with Factor IV is higher than with Factor VIII, but these reactions are usually mild.
3. See Special Nursing Interventions in the section on whole blood for notes on AIDS.

4. Antibodies to the AIDS virus have been detected in hemophiliac patients treated with Factor VIII and Factor IX concentrates (Gjerset et al, 1985; Gjerset et al, 1984; Levy et al, 1984); careful screening of all donated blood products should help decrease the risk of AIDS transmission.
5. The National Hemophilia Foundation Medical and Scientific Advisory Council, in their *Medical Bulletin #15*, October 13, 1984, listed recommendations for the prevention of AIDS in hemophiliacs, including the use of heat-treated factor concentrates that have had the AIDS virus inactivated during the manufacturing process (Rutman and Miller, 1985).
6. Additional studies have supported the use of licensed heat-treated antihemophilic factor to reduce the risk of AIDS transmission (Levy et al, 1985; McDougal et al, 1985, Petricciani et al, 1985).

Albumin (5% and 25%) and Plasma Protein Fraction (PPF)

Description and Shelf Life

1. Albumin is a chemically processed fraction of pooled plasma; 5% albumin is available in 250-ml and 500-ml amounts, and 25% albumin is available in 50-ml and 100-ml amounts.
2. PPF is a similar preparation that contains albumin and α- and β-globulins; it is available in 250-ml and 500-ml amounts.
3. Both albumin and PPF contain no blood group antigens or coagulation factors and have been heat treated during manufacture to inactivate viruses; both can be stored below 30°C for 3 years.

Indications for Use

1. Treatment of hemorrhagic shock due to trauma, infection, surgery, or burns
2. Adult respiratory distress syndrome, cerebral edema, hypoalbuminemia, acute liver failure, ascites

Equipment Recommendations

1. Recommendations are the same as for whole blood, but usually the set provided with the product is used.
2. A smaller-gauge needle may be used.

Administration Techniques

1. Usually only one person is needed for identification of product and patient.
2. Undiluted 25% albumin usually is given at a slow rate of 1 ml/min (no more than 2 ml–3 ml/min) to patients with normal blood volume to prevent rapid expansion of plasma volume and consequent fluid overload.
3. In the treatment of shock an initial dose of 100 ml to 200 ml of 25% albumin is infused as rapidly as can be tolerated by the patient.

Special Nursing Interventions

1. ABO group and Rh type compatibility are unnecessary because albumin and PPF contain no blood group antigens or antibodies.
2. Usually, 5% albumin or PPF is given to patients who need intravascular volume expansion during dehydration; 25% albumin is used for patients who need intravascular volume but also have extravascular fluid accumulation.
3. Infuse 25% albumin with extreme caution and monitor patients diligently for signs of fluid overload of pulmonary edema since large amounts of fluid will be pulled into circulation rapidly.
4. Albumin and PPF carry virtually no risk of hepatitis or AIDS transmission, since they are heat treated during the manufacturing process.

$Rh_0(D)$ Immune Globulin (RhIG)

Description and Shelf Life

1. Immune anti-D preparations in the United States contain approximately 300 μg of antibody per milliliter.
2. These preparations can be stored for 18 months at 2°C to 8°C.

3. A 1-ml dose is sufficient to counteract the immunizing effects of 15 ml of Rh-positive red cells. (This corresponds to 30 ml of fetal blood.)

Indications for Use

1. RhIG is given to Rh-negative persons who receive Rh-positive erythrocytes through either accidental transfusion (such as during platelet or granulocyte administration), pregnancy (including miscarriage, abortion, or other pregnancy outcomes), or following amniocentesis or other abnormal trauma during pregnancy to prevent active immunization against the Rh antigen.

Equipment Recommendations

1. RhIG is usually given by intramuscular (IM) injection.

Administration Techniques

1. RhIG should be administered intramuscularly to an Rh-negative woman as soon as possible after or within 72 hours of delivery of an Rh-positive infant.
2. RhIG should also be given following amniocentesis or after miscarriage, abortion, or other pregnancy outcomes unless the father is known to be Rh negative.
3. Dosage is usually based on the quantity of RBCs that were infused. (Usually a dose of one vial containing 300 μg of antibody is adequate.)
4. Many investigators feel that RhIG should be given not only at delivery but also at 28 weeks' gestation for complete protection during pregnancy.

Special Nursing Interventions

1. Compatibility between RBCs of the patient and RhIG is unnecessary.
2. Following IM injection expect some tenderness at the site and a slight elevation of temperature.
3. Recent studies have shown that therapeutic immune globulin preparations carry no discernible risk of

transmitting HTLV-III/LAV infection and that current indications for their clinical use should not be changed based on such concerns (Safety of therapeutic immune globulin preparations, CDC, 1986)

Administration Procedures for Blood and Blood Products

1. Perform a patient assessment before the transfusion.
   - Patient history
     Review disease or injury states that might affect the transfusion.
     Review the transfusion history and report to the physician and blood bank any history of adverse reaction during or after any previous blood transfusion.
     Check for any drug allergies and note any medications the patient is currently receiving.
   - Review of laboratory reports
     Hemoglobin and hematocrit
     Blood grouping and cross match results
     Hepatitis testing
   - Patient education
     Make sure the patient understands the need for transfusion and what therapeutic results can be expected.
     Explain the transfusion procedure carefully to the patient and ask him to immediately report any adverse reactions he may experience during the procedure.
     Be prepared to discuss the patient's fears concerning AIDS.
     If a consent form is required, make sure it is signed before the start of the transfusion.
2. Assemble all needed equipment.
   - Needle or plastic catheter
     Use an 18- or 19-gauge needle or plastic catheter for most adults.
     Use a 21-, 22-, or 23-gauge needle or plastic catheter for infants and children, geriatric patients,

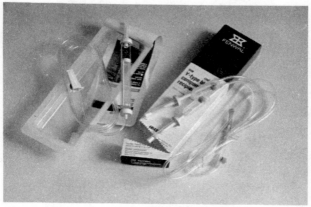

Figure 15-1. Blood administration set.

or adults who are dehydrated or are on long-term IV therapy, chemotherapy, or radiation therapy.

· Administration set (Fig. 15-1)

A Y set is recommended because it decreases the risk of contamination, allows administration of additional products safely and easily, and allows addition of normal saline to packed RBCs to decrease viscosity (Fig. 15-2).

Use the proper administration set for the component being infused.

A single administration set may be used for transfusion of 2 to 4 units; it is usually recommended that both the unit of blood and the administration set not remain in use for more than 4 hours.

· Filter (Fig. 15-3)

All blood products must be given through tubing that contains an in-line blood filter (pore size 170 μ).

These standard blood filters are available with either a regular-size surface area or a large-size

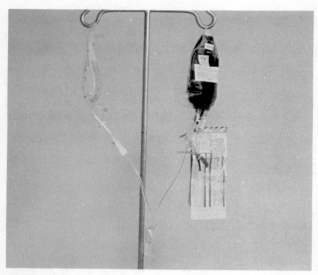

Figure 15-2. Y set.

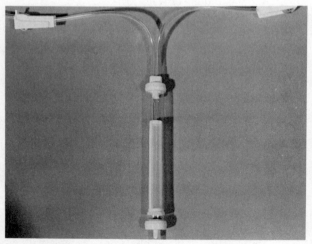

Figure 15-3. Standard blood filter.

surface area (for transfusing 2–4 units of blood or transfusing at a faster rate).

Microaggregate filters (pore size 20 μ–40 μ) are available for use with patients who may require increased filtering of transfused blood to decrease debris and clots that might otherwise lodge in their alveoli and inhibit pulmonary function (these patients might be neonates, those with compromised pulmonary status, or multiple-unit recipients); most microaggregate filters may be used for 3 to 6 units of blood before they are changed, but be sure to check with each filter manufacturer for specific recommendations.

· Pumping device

Infusion pumps specifically for blood transfusion may be used.

Pressure sleeves that maintain pressure up to 300 mm Hg may be used.

· Warming device

Blood-warming coils or electrical warming systems may be used when infusing large amounts of blood rapidly through a central venous pressure line.

To prevent hemolysis, blood should never be warmed to a temperature higher than 37°C.

· Blood or blood product

Follow the institution's guidelines for ordering and obtaining blood.

Do not obtain the blood until just before giving it; blood that is outside of the blood bank–monitored refrigerator for more than 30 minutes cannot be returned to the blood bank.

3. Identify the patient and the blood product (Fig. 15-4).

· Follow the institution's guidelines for identification procedures.

In most institutions at least two persons are required to identify patient and blood product (Fig. 15-5).

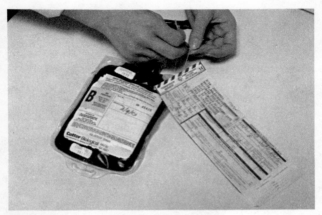

Figure 15-4. Blood product identification.

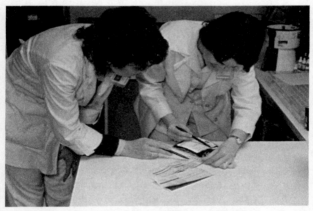

Figure 15-5. Two persons identify patient and blood product.

- Blood product identification

  Check the blood bag compatibility tag against the order on the patient's chart.

  Check the expiration date on the blood tag.

  Check the blood product closely for any clots, discoloration, hemolysis, or bubbles.

- Patient identification

  If the patient is responsive ask him to state his full name.

  If the patient is unresponsive, a family member can give the patient's name.

  Check the patient's wristband and the identification numbers on the transfusion wristband for correspondence with those on the compatibility tag on the blood bag.

- *Remember:* most major transfusion reactions result from clerical and identification errors!

4. Take baseline vital signs of the patient before the transfusion is started.

5. Begin the transfusion *slowly.*

   - Use only normal saline to prime the line (0.9% sodium chloride).

     Do not use 5% dextrose in water.

     Do not use calcium-containing solutions such as lactated Ringer's.

   - Adjust the transfusion rate to approximately 2 ml/min.

     Allow no more than approximately 30 ml to be transfused during that first 15-minute period.

     Watch the patient carefully and continuously during the first 15 minutes. If any adverse reactions occur the transfusion can be stopped and only a small amount of blood will have been transfused. (See Tables 15-1 and 15-2 for signs and symptoms of transfusion reactions.)

     Take the patient's vital signs several times during the first 15 minutes.

   - If no adverse reactions have occurred, maintain the ordered transfusion rate (Fig. 15-6).

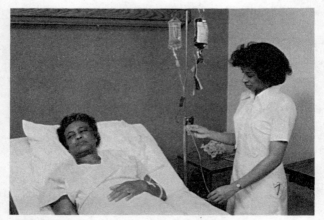

Figure 15-6. Maintain ordered transfusion rate.

The entire unit should be transfused within 2 hours but can take up to 4 hours.

Monitor the patient often during the transfusion.

Agitate the blood product gently several times during the transfusion.

• If an adverse reaction occurs, follow the institution's transfusion reaction procedures. (See Tables 15-1 and 15-2 for information about transfusion reactions.)

Notify the physician and the blood bank.

Return all parts of the administration set and blood product to the laboratory as ordered.

Collect blood and urine samples from the patient as ordered.

Treat the patient for complications as ordered.

Document necessary information following the transfusion reaction according to institutional protocol.

6. Follow institutional documentation procedures during and following the transfusion.

• Person(s) performing transfusion

- Specific product(s) administered
- Patient's baseline vital signs before and during transfusion
- Times transfusion was started and finished
- Response of patient during the transfusion
- Any nursing action taken during the transfusion
- Total amount of fluid transfused (including starter solution)

Complications

Tables 15-1 and 15-2 summarize the possible transfusion reactions seen in administration of blood and blood products.

Table 15-1. Transfusion Reactions With an Immunologic Basis

Type of Reaction	Cause	Onset

Febrile (nonhemolytic)
   Most common reaction
   Seen mostly in multitransfused and multiparous patients
	Recipient anti-HLA antibodies react with donor granulocytes, platelets, and lymphocytes	Can occur immediately or within 1–2 hours after transfusion

Allergic (mild)
   Second most common reaction
   Usually not serious
   Seen more with granulocytes and plasma than with RBCs
	Due to soluble allergens in blood product	Can occur immediately or within 1 hour after transfusion

Delayed hemolytic
   Fairly common reaction but frequently missed
   Seen in multitransfused and multiparous patients
	1°: patient exposed to foreign RBC antigen by pregnancy or transfusion, produces antibodies	1°: 10–14 days after transfusion

Clinical Signs and Symptoms	Nursing Interventions	Prevention
Fever, with or without shaking chills Headache Nausea, vomiting Hypotension Chest pain Nonproductive cough, dyspnea Malaise, myalgia No hemoglobinemia or hemoglobinuria	Stop transfusion Keep vein open Notify physician Monitor vital signs p.r.n. Keep patient warm Aspirin or acetaminophen as ordered by physician (antihistamines of no value)	Give leukocyte-poor blood and blood products to patients with prior reactions (washed RBCs or frozen deglycerolized RBCs) Give HLA-compatible blood and blood products
No fever Skin involvement: Itching, hives, local erythema, rash, urticaria Discomfort Anxiety	Stop transfusion but keep vein open; check for possible clerical error—if none found and no other symptoms develop, slowly resume transfusion Administer antihistamines as ordered by physician Monitor vital signs p.r.n.	Give antihistamines prior to transfusion (*do not* mix antihistamines in blood product!)
1°: Most go unnoticed May have decreasing hemoglobin level Positive direct antiglobulin test	Notify physician Majority of cases do not need treatment	Use sensitive antibody identification methods before transfusion If 48 hours have passed since last transfusion, re–cross match

Continued

Table 15-1. (Continued)

Type of Reaction	Cause	Onset
Delayed hemolytic, *cont.* Most are not serious	2°: anamnestic response following exposure to same foreign antigen	2°: 1–5 days after transfusion
Acute hemolytic Uncommon but potentially life-threatening Caused by clerical error more often than cross match error Usually dose related; can occur with less than 30 ml blood	ABO group incompatibility	Usually occurs during first 15 minutes of transfusion, but can occur at any time during transfusion

Clinical Signs and Symptoms	Nursing Interventions	Prevention
2°: Fever Anemia Mild jaundice Purpura Positive direct antiglobulin test		
Fever, flushing, chills Increased pulse rate Lumbar pain Hypotension Nausea and vomiting Headache Chest pain, dyspnea Hemoglobinemia/hemoglobinuria Oliguria/anuria Abnormal bleeding Shock Disseminated intravascular coagulation (DIC)	Stop transfusion Keep vein open Notify physician Check for possible clerical error Monitor vital signs p.r.n. Assess for signs and symptoms of shock Maintain intravascular volume with colloids or crystalloids as ordered Prevent renal vasoconstriction with diuretics or mannitol; monitor urine output; give dopamine as ordered by physician Collect blood and urine samples for lab and blood bank	Follow identification procedures *to the letter* for patient and blood product Start transfusion slowly and stay with the patient during the first 15 minutes of transfusion Monitor patient closely during transfusion for any adverse reactions

Continued

Table 15-1. (Continued)

Type of Reaction	Cause	Onset
Allergic (anaphylactic) Very rare but potentially life-threatening	Patients with congenital deficiency of IgA are sensitized during pregnancy of transfusion; at next transfusion immediate antigen–antibody complexes form and activate complement cascade; shock results	Rapid onset—within minutes of starting transfusion

Graft vs host disease
  Occurs in immunodeficient patients (children, patients following bone marrow transplant or cytotoxic drug therapy, fetuses after intrauterine transfusion)
  Rare, but can progress to fatal outcome
	Immunocompetent donor lymphocytes engraft and replicate, react against "foreign" tissues of the recipient	Varies with clinical situation

Clinical Signs and Symptoms	Nursing Interventions	Prevention
Flushing, dyspnea, wheezing, decrease in BP, shock GI distress: vomiting, nausea, cramping, diarrhea No fever Anxiety Arrest/death	Stop transfusion Keep vein open Notify physician Monitor vital signs every 15 minutes Maintain intravascular volume and BP with crystalloid by physician Administer epinephrine, steroids, and dopamine as ordered by physician Begin resuscitative measures p.r.n.	Transfuse patients with anaphylactic history with IgA-deficient blood products: washed RBCs or frozen deglycerolized RBCs
Fever Hepatitis Diarrhea Bone marrow suppression Infection Lymphadenopathy Hepatosplenomegaly Hemolytic anemia Pancytopenia	Assess signs and symptoms	Transfuse immunodeficient patients with washed RBCs or lymphocyte-containing blood products that have been irradiated as ordered by physician

Table 15-2. Transfusion Reactions With a Nonimmunologic Basis

Type of Reaction	Cause	Onset
Bacterial contamination Occurs rarely owing to high standards of donor blood collection techniques, adequate refrigeration standards, and adherence to aseptic technique during transfusion	Bacteria introduced into blood product or blood transfusion delivery system; bacterial endotoxins cause sepsis and shock in blood recipient	Can occur immediately or within 1 hour after transfusion
Circulatory overload More common with whole blood, but excessive volume of any component can be implicated Frequently seen in elderly, children, and heart patients	Too rapid an infusion or too great a volume of blood is given to a patient prone to circulatory overload	Can occur at any time during transfusion or following several transfusions in a short period

Clinical Signs and Symptoms	Nursing Interventions	Prevention
High fever with chills Abdominal cramping Vomiting Diarrhea Flushed dry skin Renal failure Hemoglobinuria DIC Shock	Stop transfusion Keep vein open Notify physician Change blood administration set, send blood and set to lab Monitor vital signs p.r.n. Administer antibiotics, steroids, vasopressors, fluids, and other drugs as ordered by physician	Use strict aseptic technique in blood collection, component preparation, transfusion procedures Always examine blood product carefully before administration for any clots, discoloration, hemolysis, or bubbles Do not return unused blood to blood bank (blood not used within 30 minutes after removal from blood bank refrigerator cannot be returned)
Dyspnea and cyanosis Dry cough Severe headache Pulmonary edema Rapid rise in systolic BP Increase in central venous pressure	Slow rate of or discontinue transfusion Sit the client up Monitor vital signs p.r.n. Use O_2, diuretics, digitalis, positive-pressure breathing, and rotating tourniquets as ordered by physician	Closely monitor patients prone to fluid overload Administer packed RBCs in place of whole blood when possible as ordered by physician Give future transfusions in smaller volumes

Continued

Table 15-2. (Continued)

Type of Reaction	Cause	Onset
Air embolism Rare, but potentially life-threatening	Air bubbles enter patient circulation, usually due to blood infusion under pressure	Can occur at any time during transfusion
Hypothermia Rare, but symptomatology can be severe although usually brief	Large amounts of blood given rapidly can reduce body temperature significantly	Within 30 minutes, 5 units of refrigerated blood may reduce body temperature to approximately 4°C
Hypocalcemia Very rare	Massive transfusion of any citrated product—citrate binds with and lowers circulating ionized calcium in the blood	Following massive transfusion (as 1 unit in 5 min or 20 units in 2 hr) or in patients with impaired liver function

Clinical Signs and Symptoms	Nursing Interventions	Prevention
Sudden onset of cough Shortness of breath Chest pain Cyanosis Hypotension Shock	Clamp off transfusion Administer O$_2$ Place client on left side with head down Treat shock or cardiac arrest as ordered by physician Monitor vital signs p.r.n.	Use care and caution in starting, priming, or changing any IV system or component
Chills Irregular pulse Cardiac arrest	Monitor client's temperature during multiple-unit transfusion Treat with warmed blood and crystalloid as ordered by physician Decrease rate of transfusion Monitor vital signs p.r.n. Be alert for possible metabolic acidosis	Transfuse warmed blood (temperature to be no higher than 37°C) for these patients: Neonates Multiple-unit transfusion recipients Patients with cold agglutinins
Tingling of extremities Carpopedal spasm Laryngeal stridor Hypotension Cardiac arrhythmias and arrest	Slow or stop transfusion Monitor ECG Administer oral or IV calcium preparations as ordered by physician	Administer washed or frozen deglycerolized RBCs to reduce amount of citrate infused from plasma as ordered by physician

Continued

Table 15-2. (Continued)

Type of Reaction	Cause	Onset
Disease transmission (can all be caused by donor blood containing the infectious agent that is transfused to the susceptible recipient)	Hepatitis B	1–6 months
	Hepatitis non-A, non-B	2–26 weeks
	Cytomegalovirus (CMV)	3–8 weeks

Clinical Signs and Symptoms	Nursing Interventions	Prevention
Abnormal liver function tests	Aimed at prevention	Careful blood donor screening
Elevated liver enzymes		Serologic detection in donor unit
Weakness		Education of medical personnel
Fatigue		
Nausea		
Jaundice		
Aversion to cigarettes		
May be no symptoms	Aimed at prevention	Careful blood donor screening
Flulike symptoms		Education of medical personnel
Icteric or nonicteric symptoms		No pretransfusion testing available
Generally a mild disease		
Can result in chronic liver disease		
Generalized infection		
Fatigue		
Weakness		
Symptoms similar to mononucleosis		
Generalized infection	Aimed at prevention	Careful blood donor screening
Fatigue		Education of medical personnel
Weakness		Testing of donor blood to isolate CMV can be done
Symptoms similar to mononucleosis		

Continued

Table 15-2. (Continued)

Type of Reaction	Cause	Onset
	Syphilis	10 days–10 weeks
	AIDS	6 months–5 years
	Malaria	12 days–2 months

Clinical Signs and Symptoms	Nursing Interventions	Prevention
Lymph node swelling	Aimed at prevention	Careful blood donor screening
Mild constitutional symptoms		Serologic detection in donor unit
Clinical latency of weeks to years		Education of medical personnel
May be occurrence of infectious lesions		
Fever	Aimed at prevention	Careful blood donor screening
Night sweats		Serologic detection in donor unit
Weight loss		
Enlargement of lymph nodes		Education of medical personnel
Opportunistic infections		Defer members of high-risk groups
Skin lesions		Education of public
Fever	Aimed at prevention	Careful blood donor screening for past history, recent travel
Chills		
Sweats		
Headache		Defer immigrants for 3 years
May progress to icterus, shock, coma, other CNS symptoms		Known carriers or persons having had malaria deferred permanently

Bibliography

Birdsall C: How do you avoid transfusion complications? Am J Nurs 85:312, 1985

Blood Transfusion Therapy, A Physician's Handbook. Arlington, VA, American Association of Blood Banks, 1983

Circular of Information for the Use of Human Blood and Blood Components. Washington, DC, American Association of Blood Banks and American Red Cross, 1981

Coolfont Report: A PHS plan for prevention and control of AIDS and the AIDS virus. Public Health Rep 101(4):341, 1986

Curran JW, Lawrence DN, Jaffe H et al: Acquired immunodeficiency syndrome (AIDS) associated with transfusions. N Engl J Med 310:69, 1984

Curran JW, Morgan WM, Hardy AM et al: The epidemiology of AIDS: Current status and future prospects. Science 229:1352, 1985

Gjerset FG, Martin PJ, Counts RB et al: Immunologic status of hemophilia patients treated with cryoprecipitate or lyophilized concentrate. *Blood* 64:715, 1984

Gjerset FG, McGrady G, Counts RB et al: Lymphadenopathy-associated virus antibodies and T cells in hemophiliacs treated with cryoprecipitate or concentrate. Blood 66:718, 1985

Guidelines to Transfusion Practices. Washington, DC, American Association of Blood Banks, 1980

Jaffe HW: The acquired immunodeficiency syndrome epidemic: Issues for health care professionals. Am J Infect Control 14(6):272, 1986

Levy JA, Mitra G, Mozen MM: Recovery and inactivation of infectious retroviruses from factor VIII concentrates. Lancet 2:722, 1984

Levy JA, Mitra G, Mozen M: Recovery of AIDS-associated retrovirus (ARV) from lyophilized factor VIII products after addition of virus to plasma (abstr 70). International Conference on Acquired Immunodeficiency Syndrome (AIDS), Atlanta, Georgia, 1985

McDougal JS, Martin LS, Cort SP et al: Thermal inactivation of the AIDS virus, LAV/HTLV-III, with special reference to antihemophilic factor. J Clin Invest 76:875, 1985

Petricciani JC, McDougal JS, Evatt BL: Letter: Case for concluding that heat-treated, licensed anti-hemophilic factor is free from HTLV-III. Lancet October 19, 1985

Pindyck J, Waldman A, Zang A et al: Measures to decrease the risk of acquired immunodeficiency syndrome transmission by blood transfusion. Transfusion 25:3, 1985

Pittiglio D: Modern Blood Banking and Transfusion Practices. Philadelphia, FA Davis, 1983

Popovsky MA: Autologous transfusion. NITA 9:292, 1986

Popovsky MA, Taswell HF: Role of I.V. and transfusion nurses in autologous transfusion. NITA 7:385, 1984

Recommendations for preventing transmission of infection with HTLV-III/LAV during invasive procedures. MMWR 35(14):221, 1986

Rutman R, Miller W: Transfusion Therapy Principles and Procedures. Baltimore, Aspen, 1985

Safe Transfusion. Washington, DC, American Association of Blood Banks, 1981

Safety of therapeutic immune globulin preparations with respect to transmission of HTLV-III/LAV infection. MMWR 35(14):231, 1986

Standards for Blood Banks and Transfusion Services. Arlington, VA, American Association of Blood Banks, 1984

Surveillance of hemophilia-associated acquired immunodeficiency syndrome. MMWR 35(43):669, 1986

Technical Manual. Arlington, VA, American Association of Blood Banks, 1985

Transfusion-associated HTLV-III/LAV from a seronegative donor. MMWR 35(24):389, 1986

Weir JA: Virus, a concern in transfusion therapy. NITA 9:234, 1986

Wells MA, Wittek A, Marcus-Sekura C et al: Chemical and physical inactivation of human T lymphotropic virus, Type III (HTLV-III). Transfusion 26:110, 1986

Zuck TF: Editorial: Comments on lessons learned this past year from HIV antibody testing and from counseling blood donors. Transfusion 26(6):493, 1986

16 ▷ Home Intravenous Therapy

Key Points

1. Indications for home IV therapy
2. Patient selection criteria
3. Vascular access methods
4. Policies and procedures
5. Patient education considerations

Indications for Home IV Therapy

Patients with certain diseases or conditions requiring long-term IV therapy are potential candidates for home IV therapy. Examples may include the following:

1. Parenteral nutrition (PN)
   - Small-bowel resection culminating in short-bowel syndrome
   - Inflammatory bowel disease
   - Pancreatitis
   - Gastrointestinal fistula
   - Congenital malabsorption syndrome
   - Scleroderma
   - Neoplastic disease
   - Various other conditions
2. Chemotherapy
   - Breast cancer
   - Hodgkin's disease
   - Lung cancer
   - Acute and chronic lymphocytic leukemia
   - Skin cancer
   - Burkitt's lymphoma

- Ovarian cancer
- Testicular cancer
- Bladder cancer
- Pancreatic cancer
- Colorectal cancer
- Various other types of cancer

3. IV antibiotics
   - Bacterial endocarditis
   - Osteomyelitis
   - Septic arthritis
   - Chronic urinary tract infections
   - Cystic fibrosis
   - Various other infections

4. Blood component therapy
   - Degenerative hepatic disease secondary to alcoholism
   - Anemic states
   - Clotting deficiencies
   - Various other conditions

5. Other IV fluids
   - Fluid replacement
   - Electrolyte replacement
   - Pain control continuous infusions
   - Various other conditions

Patient Selection Criteria

Before a patient can be selected as a candidate for home IV therapy, he should be evaluated as follows:

1. Physical and emotional state, and anticipated psychosocial effects of home IV therapy
2. Type and duration of therapy that will be needed
3. Availability of appropriate IV delivery system for the home setting and patient's need and abilities
4. Willingness of the patient/family/significant other to accept home therapy
5. Patient's ability to handle the home-care responsibilities

- Manual dexterity
- Ability to see well
- Educability
- Compliance
- Motivation
6. Availability of family member or friend to help with the patient's care if necessary
7. Home environment
   - Electricity and proper plumbing present
   - Adequate heating/air conditioning
   - Refrigerator/freezer available if necessary
   - Storage space available
   - General cleanliness
   - Telephone present
8. Individual reimbursement capabilities

Vascular Access Methods

To select a vascular access device, the physician must evaluate the type and duration of therapy that will be needed and also consider patient capabilities and preferences. The following types of vascular access devices are available:

1. Peripheral catheter, including heparin lock and continuous peripheral infusion—see Chapters 3, 5, and 6 for a discussion of these devices
2. Subclavian catheter—see Chapter 11
3. Peripherally inserted central catheter—see Chapter 11
4. Hickman, Broviac, or Groshong catheter—see Chapter 11
5. Totally implantable venous access ports—see Chapter 11

Policies and Procedures

Policies and procedures for home IV therapy should not differ from the ones followed in the hospital. Ideas for policies and procedures that should be established specifically for home IV therapy might include the following:

1. Patient qualifications
   - Disease process responding to treatment
   - Patient afebrile for at least 3 days prior to going home
2. Patient education
   - Before discharge, patient must demonstrate a thorough knowledge of all aspects of his care, including demonstration of equipment use
3. Cooperation with support services
   - Pharmacist
   - Physician
   - Visiting nurse
   - Provider of medical supplies/equipment
4. Catheter care (see Chapters 5, 6, and 11)
5. Heparin use (see Chapters 7 and 11)
6. Use of mechanical controlling devices (see Chapter 3)
7. Documentation (see Chapter 6)
8. Consent forms, if necessary
   - Blood component therapy
   - Certain medication protocols
   - Complication consequences
9. Patient monitoring, including possible complications (see Chapters 8, 9, 11, and 12)
10. Legal considerations (see Chapter 18)
    - Develop institutional standards of care
    - Refer to published standards of care (NITA, 1986; NITA, 1982; Simmons, 1982; Wiseman, 1985)
11. Training and in-service requirements for hospital/health-care agency personnel

Patient Education Considerations

Patients as well as family members must be instructed in the care and management of home IV therapy before the patient can be discharged from the hospital. During the educational sessions, patient self-confidence must be promoted. The educator should assess the learning capability and level of the patient and use effective teaching styles to present the material. Patients (and family members) must be able to demonstrate proficiency in performing and understanding all important aspects of the program before their discharge.

Topics to include in the educational program are the following:

1. Handwashing and aseptic technique
2. Operation of all equipment, including "hands on" demonstration of equipment operation
3. Care of catheter and insertion site, including hands on demonstration of site and catheter care
4. How to recognize possible complications associated with IV therapy, and steps to take if complications occur; emergency procedures
5. All aspects of the medication/solution to be given—dosage, side-effects, storage requirements, incompatibilities, administration procedure, expiration dates
6. Troubleshooting and problem-solving techniques for technical problems
7. Proper care of disposable equipment
8. How and when to contact the hospital or home health agency
   • Phone numbers
   • Contact person(s)
   • Hours of operation
   • How and where to obtain extra equipment/solutions

Bibliography

Beck ML, Grindon AJ: Home transfusion therapy. Transfusion 26(3):296, 1986

Blackburn GL, Baptista RJ: Home TPN: State of the art. Am J Intravenous Ther Clin Nutr, pp 20–32, February 1984

Bledsoe L: Discharge planning for the home care I.V. patient. NITA 8:486, 1985

Duval A, Hennessy K: Care of the Broviac catheter. NITA 6:40, 1983

Fisher W: Complication of a Hickman catheter: Cutaneous erosion of the Dacron cuff. JAMA 254:2934, 1985

Ford R: History and organization of the Seattle-area Hickman catheter committee. NITA 8:123, 1985

Gardner C: Home I.V. therapy, part I. NITA 9:95, 1986

Gardner C: Home I.V. therapy, part II. NITA 9:193, 1986

Koithan M: Home total parenteral nutrition complications. NITA 8:231, 1985

Miller PC: Home blood component therapy. NITA 9:213, 1986

National Intravenous Therapy Association: Standards for home I.V. therapy. NITA Update 7(1):2, 1986

National Intravenous Therapy Association: Standards of Practice. NITA 5:19, 1982

Rehm SJ, Weinstein AJ: Home intravenous antibiotic therapy: A team approach. Ann Intern Med 99:388, 1983

Schaffner A: Safety precautions in home chemotherapy. Am J Nurs, pp 346–347, March 1984

Sheehan K, Gildea J: Home antibiotic therapy: A less-than-ideal candidate. NITA 8:157, 1985

Simmons BP: Guidelines for the prevention of intravascular infections: Guidelines for the prevention and control of nosocomial infections. NITA 5:40, 1982

Teich CJ, Raia K: Teaching strategies for an ambulatory chemotherapy program. Oncology Nurs Forum 11(5):24, 1984

Whatley K et al: Developing a patient assessment and teaching program for right atrial catheters. NITA 7:529, 1984

Wilkes G et al: Long-term venous access. Am J Nurs, pp 793–796, July 1985

Winters V: Implantable vascular access devices. Oncology Nurs Forum 11(6):25, 1984

Wiseman M: Setting standards for home I.V. therapy. Am J Nurs, pp 421–423, April 1985

Unit VI

Promoting Safety for the Intravenous Therapy Practitioner

17 ▷ Occupational Hazards Associated With Intravenous Therapy

Key Points

1. Physical hazards
2. Infectious hazards
3. Psychosocial hazards

Physical Hazards

It is well documented that hospitals can be hazardous places for patients (Jemison-Smith and Gallagher, 1985; Gallagher and Jemison-Smith, 1985). Hospitals also may be very hazardous for the people who work in them (Clever, 1981; Omenn and Morris, 1984), and this includes personnel who administer IV therapy.

Accidents: Needle Sticks

Causes

1. Recapping needle
2. Improperly discarding used needle in container
3. Bending, cutting, or breaking needles during disposal
4. Accidental needle sticks while performing tasks
5. Improperly transporting used needles
6. Carelessness

Risks

There is a risk of disease transmission. Hepatitis B and herpetic whitlow are most often reported, but transmission of acquired immunodeficiency syndrome (AIDS), malaria, varicella zoster virus infection, and Rocky Mountain spotted fever have all been reported following needle sticks (Sumner, 1985; McCray, 1986; Weiss et al, 1985).

Prevention
1. Do not bend, break, cut, or recap needles after use.
2. Dispose of needles in rigid, puncture-resistant, leak-proof containers that will eventually be incinerated or autoclaved; have these containers accessible at key locations (Recommendations for preventing HTLV-III/LAV, 1986; Jemison-Smith and Hamm, 1985; Crow, 1985).

Accidents: Abrasions and Contusions

Causes
Abrasions and contusions are caused by contact with broken glass, sharp edges of containers, or almost any sharp or jagged-edged item.

Risks
Small or undetected skin abrasions or contusions can be portals of entry for microorganisms such as *Staphylococcus aureus, Herpes simplex,* and the AIDS virus; cellulitis or deeper infection can result.

Prevention
1. Use care when assembling and manipulating IV equipment and performing other tasks.
2. Use excellent handwashing technique.
3. Cover small abrasions or cuts with a Band-Aid or other small bandage to protect and prevent infection.

Radiation Exposure

Causes
Most radiation absorbed by hospital personnel is in the form of low linear energy transfer radiation, mainly as a result of the scatter of x-ray beams or the emission of gamma rays (Zeimer and Orvis, 1981); exposures can occur in the radiology department or in nuclear medicine,

from portable x-ray equipment, from patient body burden of radionucleotides, and from hospital waste (Nuclear Medicine, 1982). Intravenous therapy personnel may be exposed to radiation during radiologic confirmation of catheter placement or when assisting IV therapy patients who are undergoing radiologic procedures.

Risks
Clinical concerns include cancer, teratogenesis, and possible genetic effects in the descendents of exposed persons.

Prevention
The most important safeguards are an aggressive radiation protection education program and the implementation of technological advances that will reduce exposures (Laughlin, 1981).

Chemical Exposure: Cytotoxic Drugs

Causes
Handling of cytotoxic (antineoplastic) drugs can be hazardous.

Risks
Nurses handling cytotoxic drugs may have urine capable of inducing mutations in bacterial systems (Falck et al, 1979) and an increased frequency of sister chromatid exchange in their peripheral lymphocytes (Norppa et al, 1980); neurologic symptoms and liver disease have been reported in three oncology nurses who lacked other causes for hepatitis (Sotaniemi et al, 1983).

Prevention
1. The use of vertical flow biologic safety cabinets can prevent urine mutagenicity (Nguyen et al, 1982).
2. Gloves, gowns, and goggles can be worn during preparation and administration of these drugs.
3. Refer to Chapter 14 for specific recommendations on

handling antineoplastic drugs and to other specific sources (OSHA, 1986).

Chemical Exposure: Handwashing Soaps

Causes

Because meticulous handwashing technique is required for all staff involved with intravenous therapy, excessive exposure to handwashing soaps may occur.

Risks

Contact dermatitis is the most common result of exposure to chemicals and is the most common occupational illness. Allergic reactions to chemicals sometimes occur and are very difficult to prevent; if product substitution is not possible, the worker should be transferred to another work area.

Prevention

1. Use mild soaps for handwashing whenever possible.
2. Use warm, not hot, water, and dry hands completely after handwashing.
3. Hand lotions are not recommended during the work shift from an infection control standpoint but may help eliminate skin dryness when used after working hours.

Infectious Hazards

Intravenous therapy nurses are constantly exposed to patients and their secretions and excretions and so are constantly exposed to infectious agents. As general recommendations for protection against occupational infections, nurses should practice excellent handwashing, consider all body secretions and fluids from patients to be potentially infectious, follow institutional infection control policies and guidelines, and comply with immunization recommendations.

Hepatitis B

Precautions
Blood and body fluid precautions are recommended for patients with hepatitis B.

Transmission
Transmission is by percutaneous or permucosal exposure to infective body fluids such as can occur in needle stick accidents and sexual exposure.

Prevention
1. Use great care in handling all body fluids and secretions from patients.
2. Use careful handling of needles and other sharp instruments.
3. Hepatitis B vaccine is recommended for all high-risk health-care workers such as IV therapy nurses.
4. Use of hepatitis B immune globulin (HBIG) is recommended after parenteral or mucosal exposure to known hepatitis-positive blood (Jemison-Smith and Hamm, 1985).

Acquired Immunodeficiency Syndrome

Precautions
Blood and body fluid precautions are recommended for patients with AIDS; other precautions depend on the patient's additional presenting illness(es).

Transmission
Transmission is by needle sticks, transfusion of blood or certain blood products, sexual contact, and IV drug abuse; the risk of nosocomial infection to health-care workers is currently reported to be very low (Henderson et al, 1986; McCray, 1986). The disease is primarily sexually transmitted and is not spread by casual contact.

Prevention
Currently no vaccine or treatment is available. Prevention in the hospital centers on using great care in handling

all body fluids and secretions from patients. The use of gloves is recommended when *any* exposure to blood or other body fluids is possible. Handle needles and other sharp instruments carefully. Members of AIDS high-risk groups should not donate blood (see Chapter 15).

Staphylococcus Aureus

Staphylococcus aureus can cause staphylococcal diseases such as carbuncles, furuncles, impetigo, abscesses, phlebitis, and septicemia.

Precautions

Contact isolation is usually recommended for infected patients; infected personnel should be evaluated by employee health service and may be removed from work.

Transmission

The primary mode of transmission is spread by hands of hospital personnel; 20% to 40% of hospital personnel carry this organism in their anterior nares.

Prevention

Emphasize handwashing procedures between patients; topical or oral antibiotics are sometimes used to treat carriers.

Psychosocial Hazards

Stress

Because the circulatory system provides such rapid access to the total organism, immediate decision-making is a necessary and integral part of providing intravenous therapy. However, it is also one that can cause a good deal of stress. In addition, the practice of IV therapy must rely on the collaborative efforts of many members of the health care team. This stressful situation is further compounded by the constant need to respond to rapid technological advances while maintaining a commitment to providing nursing services within the context of a caring philosophy.

Types
1. Organizational stress
   - Decision-making pressures
     Critical decisions must be made rapidly
     Life or death component of the decision
   - Interruptions during the work day
     impair concentration
     Often emotionally unsettling
   - Shift work and prolonged work schedules
     Disruption of circadian rhythms
     Sleep deprivation
2. Affective stress
   - Relationships with patients and fellow employees
     Dealing with a patient's death
     Dealing with conflicts
   - Job burnout
   - Avoidance behaviors
   - Depression

Manifestations
1. Denial and suppression
2. Disassociation from feelings
3. Anger and frustration
4. Avoidance behaviors
   - Sleeping late to miss work
   - Reluctance to accept responsibility
   - Emotional withdrawal
5. Frank and obvious impairment
   - Substance abuse
   - Mental illness
   - Abuse of patients

Prevention
1. Optimize shift work schedules
2. Provide adequate numbers of personnel

3. Promote teamwork
4. Provide psychological support
5. Provide intellectual support

Bibliography

Advisory Committee on Immunization Practices: Rubella prevention. MMWR 33:301–308, 1984

Advisory Committee on Immunization Practices: Varicella zoster immune globulin for the presence of chickenpox. MMWR 33:84, 1984

Clever LH: Health hazards of hospital personnel. West J Med 135:162, 1981

Crow S: Disposable needle and syringe containers. Infect Control 6(1):41, 1985

Falck K, Grohn P, Sorsa M et al: Mutagenicity in urine of nurses handling cytostatic drugs. Lancet 1:1251, 1979

Gallagher M, Jemison-Smith P: Prevalent nosocomial pathogens, part 2. NITA 8:213, 1985

Henderson DK, Saah AJ, Zak BJ et al: Risk of nosocomial infection with human T-cell lymphotropic virus type III/lymphadenopathy-associated virus in a large cohort of intensively exposed health care workers. Ann Intern Med 104:644, 1986

Jemison-Smith P, Gallagher M: Prevalent nosocomial pathogens, part 1. NITA 8:144, 1985

Jemison-Smith P, Hamm P: Preventing hepatitis B. NITA 8:283, 1985

Laughlin JS: Experience with a sustained policy of radiation safety in a nuclear medicine department. Health Phys 38:399, 1981

McCray E: Occupational risk of the acquired immunodeficiency syndrome among health care workers. N Engl J Med 314(17):1127, 1986

Nguyen TV, Theiss JC, Matney TS: Exposure of pharmacy personnel to mutagenic antineoplastic drugs. Cancer Res 42:4792, 1982

Norppa H, Sorsa M, Vainio H et al: Increased sister chromatid exchange frequencies in lymphocytes of nurses handling cytostatic drugs. Scand J Work Environ Health 6:299, 1980

Nuclear Medicine—Factors Influencing the Choice and Use of Radionucleotides in Diagnosis and Therapy, NCRP Report No. 70. Bethesda, National Council on Radiation Protection and Measurements, 1982

Omenn GS, Morris SL: Occupational hazards to health care workers: Report of a conference. Am J Ind Med 6:129, 1984

OSHA work-practice guidelines for personnel dealing with cyto-toxic (antineoplastic) drugs. Am J Hosp Pharm 43:1193, 1986

Recommendations for preventing transmission of infection with human T-lymphotropic virus type III/lymphadenopathy-associated virus in the workplace. MMWR 34:682, 691, 1985

Recommendations for preventing transmission of infection with HTLV-III/LAV during invasive procedures. MMWR 35(14):221, 1986

Sotaniemi EA, Sutinen S, Arranto AJ: Liver damage in nurses handling cytostatic agents. Acta Med Scand 214:181, 1983

Sumner W: Needlecaps to prevent needlestick injuries. Infect Control 6(12):495, 1985

Weiss SH, Saxinger WC, Rechtman D et al: HTLV-III infection among health care workers. JAMA 254(15):2089, 1985

Zeimer PL, Orvis AL: Hospital radiation safety. In Stanley PE (ed): CRC Handbook of Hospital Safety, pp 275–343. Boca Raton, FL, CRC Press, 1981

18 ▷ Quality Assurance in Intravenous Therapy

Key Points

1. Quality assurance process
2. Legal aspects of IV therapy
3. IV therapy teams
4. Resources

Since approximately 17 to 24 million hospitalized patients each year experience at least one intravascular device insertion, concern for minimizing the risks and ensuring the safety of this therapy is paramount (NITA, 1986). Some of the statistics describing these risks include the following:

1. Each year 1.3 million patients experience IV infusion phlebitis (Turco, 1983).
2. Each year 35,000 patients experience septicemia (Turco, 1983).
3. Each year 3,000 patients die as a result of complications related to blood products (Turco, 1983).
4. About 20 persons handle an IV system and its components before it reaches the patient.

A perusal of the phenomenal growth in medical malpractice claims further intensifies concern for ensuring safety. Risk management is essential. Maintaining or ensuring quality involves an understanding of the quality assurance process, standards of practice, legal aspects of IV therapy, IV therapy teams, and educational preparation in the clinical specialty of IV therapy.

Quality Assurance

Definition Process

Quality assurance is "an ongoing process that pursues and achieves a desired and feasible level of patient care according to the standards of established practice" that are instituted by the profession providing the care (Gurevich, 1983).

Key Characteristics of the Quality Assurance Process

1. Concurrent—taking place during the patient's presence
2. Periodic
3. Observable
4. Measurable

Goals of Quality Assurance

1. To prevent complications
2. To decrease morbidity/mortality
3. To decrease cost
4. To shorten hospital stay
5. To increase patient comfort

Approaches to Quality Assurance

1. Structures. This includes evaluation of the resources available, including IV nursing job descriptions, committees for development of IV policies and procedures, and patient charting forms. Guidelines used for evaluative purposes include the following:
   - Guidelines for Prevention of Intravascular Infections (available from the Centers for Disease Control and published in the January/February 1982 issue of the NITA journal)
   - National Intravenous Therapy Association (NITA) Standards of Practice (available from the national office and published in the January/February 1982 issue of the NITA journal)

- National Intravenous Therapy Association (NITA) Standards of Practice for Hyperalimentation (available from the national office and published in the March/April 1981 issue of the NITA journal)
- National Intravenous Therapy Association (NITA) Standards of Practice related to Home IV Therapy (available from the national office and published in the January/February 1986 issue of *NITA Update*).
- Joint Commission on Accreditation of Hospitals (JCAH) performance standards for IV therapy (available from JCAH)
- American Association of Blood Banks (AABB)
- Federal Drug Administration (FDA)
2. Process. This includes evaluation of the actual performance of IV procedures. Compliance with accepted standards and guidelines is evaluated.
3. Outcomes. This includes evaluation of the final results of IV therapy, including patient recovery and rates of complications.

Quality Assurance and Product Evaluation

Quality assurance includes product evaluation according to specific criteria. This evaluation process should include input from staff nurses and IV therapists, as well as purchasing managers.

1. Suggested areas for evaluation of the cannula/catheter are as follows (Grabbe, 1983):
   - Packaging
   - Sterility
   - Labeling
   - Available sizes
   - Needle guard
   - Radiopacity
   - Catheter rigidity and flexibility
   - Catheter sharpness
   - Ease with which catheter is held

- Presence of blood return chamber
- Ease in taping
2. Suggested areas for evaluation of filters are as follows (Gurevich, 1984):
   - Membrane material
   - Pore size
   - Venting characteristics
   - Flow qualities without pump
   - Psi rating
   - Connection mechanism for securing within tubing system
   - Recommended length of time for use
   - Cost
3. Suggested areas for evaluation of pumps and controllers are as follows (Storc, 1984):
   - Range of solution/medication applicability
   - Volumetric accuracy
   - Type of alarm system (*e.g.,* visual or audible)
   - Weight and portability
   - Automatic conversion to KVO rate following volume infusion
   - Electrical safety features
   - Operating instructions
   - Economical/cost-effective
   - Ease in servicing

Problem Reporting in IV Therapy

Problems or concerns with quality, performance, or safety of devices can be reported to the Practitioner Reporting System (PRS), 12601 Twinbrook Parkway, Rockville, MD 20852. Provide the following information:

1. Reporter's name
2. Hospital name, address, and phone number
3. Product name
4. Lot number, expiration date
5. Model/serial number
6. Manufacturer's name and address
7. Brief description of problem(s)

Legal Aspects of IV Therapy

1. The legal rights related to IV therapy practices are outlined within the following:
   - Nurse practice acts
   - Joint policy statements
   - Institution or agency policies
2. The concept of a "reasonably prudent IV therapist" is the measure used to identify legal sufficiency of performance.
3. Types of law applicable to IV therapy are the following:
   - *Criminal law.* An offense against the public due to its harmful effect on the welfare of society as a whole; conviction results in fine/imprisonment.
   - *Civil law.* An offense against the legal rights of a private person, property, or corporation; if harm is demonstrated, damages must be paid to the injured party.

     Tort. Private wrong by action or omission; negligence is one type.

     Malpractice (one type of negligence). Negligent conduct of a professional; failure to act in a reasonably prudent manner that results in harm to person or property
4. The most common errors in IV therapy practice involve the following:
   - Administration of medication—incorrect dosage, incorrect time of administration, administration when contraindicated
   - Failure in communication (*e.g.,* charting, orders)
   - Use of equipment—error in technique, using defective equipment, allowing another to act in an unsafe manner
   - Failure to act
5. Nursing interventions to avoid or minimize lawsuits follow:
   - Maintain a caring therapeutic relationship.
   - Observe signs and symptoms and take prompt action.

- Use all equipment properly.
- Know and follow legal guidelines of practice.
- Ensure compliance with institutional policies and procedures.
- Provide patient instruction.
- Ascertain patient's consent for or refusal of care:
  Note the patient's capacity for decision making.
  Provide reasonable information.
  Allow the patient to act voluntarily.
- Maintain confidentiality.
- Ensure completeness of the physician's orders.
- Document care in a legible, objective, and complete manner.
- Document all attempts for venipuncture, including the site of venipuncture and the client's response.

IV Therapy Teams

Intravenous teams, by specializing in delivery of IV therapy, can create quality delivery systems and have a significant impact on decreasing the complications due to IV therapy. Hospitals with IV teams consistently achieve lower rates of therapy complications, thus reducing hospital costs and length of patient stay (Chrystal, 1985; Termeer, 1985).

IV Therapy Orientation Program

The basic nursing curriculum does not prepare the graduate nurse fully for assuming IV therapy responsibilities. A comprehensive IV therapy orientation program should include advanced knowledge and skill application in the following areas (Baldwin, 1986):

1. Historical and legal aspects of IV therapy
2. Fluid and electrolyte balance
3. Communication and documentation
4. Principles of infection control
5. Administration of IV solutions
6. Venipuncture techniques

7. Principles of drug administration
8. Central venous catheters
9. Total parenteral nutrition
10. Blood component therapy
11. Pediatric IV therapy
12. Special considerations: shunts, arterial lines, quality assurance, home IV therapy

Certification of IV Therapy Personnel

Definition

Certification, as a process of recognizing that a licensed professional has met and continues to maintain specific standards in a specialty area, can be conducted by an agency or association. The National Intravenous Therapy Association (NITA) sponsors an examination that must be passed before a person may become certified. In this case, certification verifies competence in the specialty area of IV therapy.

Process

The credentialing process of NITA leading to certification involves the following steps:

1. Eligibility
2. Application
3. Validation
4. Examination
5. Certification (documentation)

Topics included on the examination are the following:

1. Fluid and electrolyte balance
2. Infection control
3. Oncology
4. Pediatrics
5. Pharmacology
6. Quality assurance
7. Technology and clinical application
8. Transfusion therapy

Individual health-care institutions can also develop certification programs. All such programs should include theory as well as clinical application components.

Resources

The following organizations can serve as resources for the safe and effective practice of IV therapy:

American Association of Critical Care Nurses
One Civic Plaza
Newport Beach, CA 92660

American Cancer Society
90 Park Avenue
New York, NY 10016

American Hospital Association
840 N. Lake Shore Drive
Chicago, IL 60611

American Nurses Association
2420 Pershing Road
Kansas City, MO 64108

Association for Practitioners in Infection Control
505 E. Hawley Street
Mundelein, IL 60060

Centers for Disease Control
Atlanta, GA 30333

National Association of Pediatric Nurse Associates and
Practitioners
1000 Maplewood Drive, Suite 104
Maple Shade, NJ 08052

National Council of State Boards of Nursing
625 N. Michigan Avenue, Suite 1544
Chicago, IL 60611

National Intravenous Therapy Association
87 Blanchard Road
Cambridge, MA 02138

Oncology Nursing Society
311 Banksville Road
Pittsburgh, PA 15216

Public Health Nursing/American Public Health Association
1015 Fifteenth Street, NW
Washington, DC 20005

Society for Peripheral Vascular Nursing
1070 Sibley Tower
Rochester, NY 14604

Bibliography

Baldwin D: Personalized system of instruction for I.V. therapy orientation. NITA 9(6):447, 1986

Bergeson S: Charting with a jury in mind. Nursing Life 2:30–37, 1982

Blust J, Henderson J: The I.V. therapist looks at the law. Am J Intravenous Ther Clin Nutr 9:12–16, 1982

Burik D, Cramton C, Holtz J: A workbook approach to justifying I.V. therapy teams under prospective payment. NITA 7:411, September/October 1984

Chrystal C: I.V. complications rates. NITA Update 6(3):5, 1985

Chrystal C: Making the NITA standards work for you. NITA 6:19, 1983

Chrystal C: Making the NITA standards work for you. NITA 6:40, January/February 1983

Chrystal C: Making the NITA standards work for you. NITA 6:89, March/April 1983

Chrystal C: Making the NITA standards work for you. NITA 6:188, May/June 1983

Chrystal C: Making the NITA standards work for you. NITA 8:363, September/October 1985

Crane V, Louviere M: I.V. therapy problem-solving with quality assurance. NITA 6:430, November/December 1983

Crudi C: Credentialing for I.V. nurses. NITA 7:233, May/June 1984

Foltz A: Evaluation of implanted infusion devices. NITA 10(1):48, 1987

Gardner C: I.V. therapy quality assurance provides risk management. NITA 8:199, May/June 1985

Grabbe M: Clinical product evaluation and proposal justification in product selection. NITA 6:268, July/August 1983

Guarriello D: Intravenous therapy and the law. NITA 6:278, July/August 1983

Gurevich I: I.V. quality assurance theory and practice. NITA 6:409, November/December 1983

Gurevich I: I.V. filters—a standard of care. NITA 7:393, September/October 1984

Hogue E: Informed consent. Nursing 86 16:47–48, 1986

Ingalls M: Expert testimony. NITA 8(6):506, 1985

Koekenberg H: Problem reporting in I.V. therapy. Infusion 8(2):47, 1984

Magel N: Quality assurance and I.V. therapy. Am J Intravenous Ther Clin Nutr 8(1):11, 1981

Mellema S, Poniatowski B: Justification of an I.V. team using productivity data. NITA 8:381, September/October 1985

Millan D: A study of I.V. therapy education. NITA 8(5):393, 1985

NITA: The importance of intravenous therapy. Health Care Decisions, September 1, 1986

Termeer J: Justification arguments. NITA Update 6(1):5, 1985

Tomford J, Huskey C: The I.V. therapy team-impact on patient care and costs of hospitalization. NITA 8:387, September/October 1985

Turco S: Clinical use of parenterals. Parenterals 1:4, 1983

Weinstein S: Expert testimony—the I.V. nurse's responsibility. NITA 7(5):423, 1984

Index

The letter *t* following a page number indicates tabular material; *f* indicates a figure.